Conquer Illness Through Nutrition: Harnessing the Power of Eating to Defeat Disease

By

Calvin M. Duncan

Table Of Contents

Chapter One

Introduction

•*The Connection Between Nutrition and Health*

The intricate connection between nutrition and health has long been recognized as a cornerstone of human well-being. As we delve into the intricate interplay between the foods we consume and our physical and mental states, it becomes clear that what we eat plays a pivotal role in shaping our overall health and vitality. This connection extends beyond mere sustenance, forming the basis of disease prevention, management, and even our longevity.

At its core, nutrition is the science that explores the relationship between the nutrients in foods and their effects on our bodies. Nutrients encompass a range of substances, from macronutrients such as carbohydrates, proteins, and fats, to micronutrients like vitamins and minerals. Each nutrient carries out specific functions within our bodies, contributing to growth, development, energy production, and immune response.

Optimal nutrition is not just about filling our stomachs; it's about providing our bodies with the essential building blocks they need to function properly. The importance of nutrition is perhaps most evident in the early stages of life. From conception to childhood, a balanced diet is crucial for proper growth and development. The nutrients obtained during these formative years lay the foundation for a lifetime of health. Inadequate nutrition during this period can lead to developmental delays, cognitive impairments, and a heightened susceptibility to diseases.

However, the impact of nutrition isn't limited to the early years. Throughout our lives, the foods we choose to consume directly influence our risk of chronic diseases. Cardiovascular diseases, such as heart disease and stroke, are among the leading causes of mortality worldwide. Research has consistently shown that diets high in saturated and trans fats, sodium, and added sugars contribute to the development of these conditions. On the other hand, diets rich in fruits, vegetables, whole grains, lean proteins, and healthy fats can substantially lower the risk of cardiovascular diseases.

Likewise, the prevalence of type 2 diabetes has surged in recent decades, largely attributed to sedentary lifestyles and poor dietary choices. Excessive consumption of sugary beverages and highly processed foods contributes to weight gain and insulin resistance, the hallmark of diabetes. By adopting a diet focused on complex carbohydrates, fiber, and lean proteins, individuals can better manage their blood sugar levels and reduce the risk of developing diabetes.

Inflammation, although a natural response of the immune system, can become chronic and contribute to a range of health problems. Poor dietary habits, characterized by high intake of refined sugars and unhealthy fats, can fuel inflammation. On the other hand, foods rich in antioxidants, omega-3 fatty acids, and phytochemicals possess anti-inflammatory properties. By incorporating these foods into our diets, we can help mitigate chronic inflammation and its associated health risks.

The gut, often referred to as the "second brain," houses a complex ecosystem of microorganisms known as the microbiome. Emerging research has underscored the pivotal role of the microbiome in maintaining not only digestive health but also influencing immunity, metabolism, and even mental health. Diets rich in fiber and diverse plant-based foods nurture a healthy microbiome, fostering a balanced composition of beneficial bacteria that can positively impact various facets of our well-being.

Mental health, an area gaining significant attention, is also intricately linked to nutrition. The gut-brain axis, a bidirectional communication network between the gut and the brain, highlights how our dietary choices can influence mood and cognitive function. Nutrients such as omega-3 fatty acids, B vitamins, and certain amino acids play a crucial role in neurotransmitter production and brain health. A diet lacking in these nutrients may contribute to conditions like depression, anxiety, and cognitive decline.

In conclusion, the connection between nutrition and health is undeniable and multifaceted. The foods we consume have a profound impact on our physical health, influencing our risk of chronic diseases and overall well-being. Nutrition isn't solely about satisfying hunger; it's about nourishing our bodies with the essential components they require to function optimally. From preventing heart disease to fostering mental resilience, our dietary choices hold the power to shape our present and future health trajectories. By understanding and harnessing the potent relationship between nutrition and health, we empower ourselves to lead longer, healthier, and more vibrant lives.

•*The Role of Food in Disease Prevention and Management*

In an era of rapid advancements in medical technology and pharmaceutical interventions, the role of food in disease prevention and management remains a vital and often underestimated aspect of healthcare. The age-old adage, "You are what you eat," holds a profound truth that resonates across cultures and generations. The intricate relationship between the foods we consume and their impact on our health is a topic of increasing importance, as both scientific research and anecdotal evidence continue to emphasize the power of nutrition in shaping our well-being.

Disease prevention, as the old saying goes, is worth a pound of cure. The foundation of disease prevention lies in maintaining a healthy lifestyle, and at the core of a healthy lifestyle is a

balanced and nutrient-dense diet. The foods we eat provide the essential nutrients that our bodies need to function optimally. These nutrients encompass a spectrum of vitamins, minerals, antioxidants, fibers, and macronutrients that work in synergy to support various bodily functions, from cellular metabolism to immune response.

One of the most striking examples of the preventive power of nutrition is the relationship between diet and cardiovascular health. Cardiovascular diseases, including heart disease and stroke, continue to be leading causes of mortality globally. However, research has consistently shown that certain dietary patterns can significantly reduce the risk of these conditions. A diet rich in fruits, vegetables, whole grains, lean proteins, and healthy fats can lower blood pressure, reduce cholesterol levels, and promote overall heart health.

Similarly, the link between nutrition and type 2 diabetes prevention is well-established. The surge in diabetes cases over the past few decades has been closely tied to changes in dietary habits and sedentary lifestyles. High intake of sugary beverages, refined carbohydrates, and unhealthy fats contributes to insulin resistance and obesity, both of which are major risk factors for diabetes. Conversely, adopting a diet that focuses on complex carbohydrates, fiber, and lean proteins can help regulate blood sugar levels and reduce the risk of developing diabetes.

Cancer, another formidable adversary to human health, also demonstrates a connection to nutrition. While genetics and environmental factors play a role in cancer development, emerging evidence points to the influence of dietary choices. Diets rich in fruits, vegetables, and whole grains provide a plethora of phytochemicals and antioxidants that have been associated with a lower risk of certain types of cancer. On the contrary, diets high in processed meats, excessive red meat, and unhealthy fats are linked to an increased risk of cancer.

The impact of nutrition extends beyond physical health; it encompasses mental and emotional well-being as well. The gut-brain connection, often referred to as the gut-brain axis, highlights the bidirectional communication between the gut and the brain. The foods we eat can influence the composition of the gut microbiome, which in turn can affect neurotransmitter production and mood regulation. Nutrients such as omega-3 fatty acids, found in fatty fish and flaxseeds, and B vitamins play a role in cognitive function and mental health. A diet lacking in these nutrients can contribute to conditions like depression and anxiety.

In the realm of disease management, nutrition plays an equally significant role. For individuals already grappling with chronic conditions, making deliberate dietary choices can help alleviate symptoms, slow disease progression, and enhance overall quality of life. Take, for instance, inflammatory conditions such as rheumatoid arthritis. Inflammation, a common factor in many chronic diseases, can be influenced by diet. Certain foods, such as those rich in omega-3 fatty acids and antioxidants, possess anti-inflammatory properties. Including these foods while minimizing pro-inflammatory substances like saturated fats and refined sugars can help manage inflammation and alleviate symptoms.

For those diagnosed with chronic kidney disease, managing dietary intake of protein, sodium, and potassium becomes paramount. By tailoring their diets to the specific needs of their bodies, individuals can help preserve kidney function and delay disease progression. Similarly, individuals with celiac disease must adopt a strict gluten-free diet to avoid triggering immune responses and damaging their intestines.

The intricate dance between nutrition and disease prevention and management demands a holistic approach. It is not merely about counting calories or restricting certain food groups. Instead, it involves understanding the complex ways in which nutrients interact with our bodies and leveraging this knowledge to make informed dietary choices.

In a world where fast food and processed snacks are readily available, making healthy choices can be challenging. However, the growing awareness of the impact of nutrition on health has paved the way for a burgeoning movement towards whole, unprocessed foods. Governments, healthcare professionals, and individuals alike are recognizing the need to prioritize nutrition in public health policies and personal routines.

In conclusion, the role of food in disease prevention and management is a profound and intricate relationship that shapes the very fabric of our well-being. From warding off cardiovascular diseases to managing chronic conditions, the foods we consume have the power to heal and protect. Harnessing this power requires education, mindfulness, and a commitment to nourishing our bodies with the nutrients they need. As we continue to unravel the mysteries of nutrition and its impact on health, one thing remains clear: the food choices we make today have the potential to influence our health and vitality far into the future.

Chapter Two

Understanding Disease-Fighting Nutrients

•*Vitamins, Minerals, and Antioxidants: Their Impact on Health*

Vitamins, minerals, and antioxidants are the unsung heroes of the nutritional world, playing essential roles in maintaining health, preventing diseases, and ensuring the proper functioning of our bodies. These micronutrients, often required in small quantities, wield a significant influence on various physiological processes. Their absence or deficiency can lead to a cascade of health issues, underscoring the critical importance of understanding their roles and ensuring their adequate intake.

Vitamins, classified as either fat-soluble (A, D, E, and K) or water-soluble (B-complex and C), are organic compounds that our bodies cannot produce in sufficient quantities and must be obtained through diet. They serve as coenzymes, facilitating various biochemical reactions that are vital for growth, metabolism, and overall well-being.

Vitamin A, for instance, plays a central role in maintaining healthy vision, immune function, and cellular differentiation. Found in foods such as carrots, sweet potatoes, and spinach, this fat-soluble vitamin is critical for the health of our skin, eyes, and mucous membranes. Vitamin D, often referred to as the "sunshine vitamin," is essential for bone health, as it promotes the absorption of calcium and phosphorus. Its deficiency has been linked to conditions like osteoporosis and a weakened immune system.

The B-complex vitamins, including B1 (thiamine), B2 (riboflavin), B3 (niacin), B6 (pyridoxine), B7 (biotin), B9 (folate), and B12 (cobalamin), are water-soluble and participate in a range of metabolic reactions. They are crucial for energy production, nerve function, DNA synthesis, and the formation of red blood cells. Folate, for instance, is vital during pregnancy as it helps prevent neural tube defects in developing fetuses. B12, on the other hand, is necessary for neurological function and the maintenance of healthy nerve cells.

Vitamin C, also known as ascorbic acid, stands out for its role as a potent antioxidant. Found in fruits like oranges, strawberries, and bell peppers, this water-soluble vitamin supports immune function, aids in wound healing, and promotes the absorption of iron from plant-based foods. Beyond these functions, vitamin C's antioxidant properties help neutralize harmful free radicals in the body, thereby contributing to the prevention of oxidative stress and associated chronic diseases.

Minerals, unlike vitamins, are inorganic elements that are essential for various bodily functions. They serve as structural components, electrolytes, and cofactors in enzymatic reactions. Calcium, the most abundant mineral in the body, is well-known for its role in maintaining strong bones and teeth. However, calcium is not alone in its significance. Magnesium, for instance, is crucial for muscle and nerve function, as well as maintaining heart rhythm. Iron is essential for oxygen transport in the blood, while zinc supports immune function and wound healing.

The impact of antioxidants on health is a testament to their ability to combat oxidative stress, a state where an imbalance between free radicals and antioxidants leads to cellular damage. This damage is implicated in the development of chronic diseases such as cardiovascular disease, cancer, and neurodegenerative disorders. Antioxidants, found in various fruits, vegetables, and whole grains, neutralize free radicals, preventing them from causing cellular harm.

Among the well-known antioxidants is vitamin E, which protects cell membranes from oxidative damage and supports skin health. Selenium, a mineral, acts as an antioxidant in enzymes that defend against oxidative stress. Polyphenols, a group of antioxidants found in foods like berries, tea, and dark chocolate, have gained attention for their potential to reduce inflammation and protect against chronic diseases.

It's important to note that while vitamins, minerals, and antioxidants offer numerous health benefits, excessive intake can also be problematic. This underscores the importance of balance and moderation in our diets. Additionally, the absorption of these micronutrients can be influenced by various factors such as age, health status, and interactions with other nutrients. For instance, vitamin D absorption is facilitated by exposure to sunlight, making it a challenge for individuals in regions with limited sunlight.

The impact of these micronutrients on health is profound and interconnected. For example, vitamin C enhances the absorption of non-heme iron (the type of iron found in plant-based foods), while vitamin D aids in calcium absorption. This interplay highlights the intricate nature of nutrient interactions and the need for a varied and balanced diet.

In conclusion, vitamins, minerals, and antioxidants are the bedrock of our health, supporting various physiological functions and protecting us from diseases. Their roles extend beyond conventional nutrition; they are vital players in our body's complex mechanisms. From promoting strong bones to defending against cellular damage, these micronutrients are instrumental in our well-being. As we navigate our dietary choices, an awareness of the importance of vitamins, minerals, and antioxidants empowers us to make informed decisions that contribute to our long-term health and vitality.

•*Essential Nutrients for Immune System Suppor*

The immune system is a complex network of cells, tissues, and organs that work together to defend the body against harmful pathogens, such as bacteria, viruses, and parasites. A strong immune system is essential for maintaining good health and preventing infections and diseases. While several factors influence immune function, proper nutrition plays a crucial role in supporting and strengthening the immune system. In this article, we will discuss the essential nutrients that are necessary for immune system support.

- Vitamin C:

Vitamin C is perhaps one of the most well-known nutrients for immune system support. It is a powerful antioxidant that helps protect immune cells from damage caused by free radicals. Vitamin C also stimulates the production of white blood cells, which are crucial for fighting off infections. Additionally, it enhances the function of various immune cells, including natural killer cells and lymphocytes.

Good food sources of vitamin C include citrus fruits (such as oranges and grapefruits), strawberries, kiwi, bell peppers, broccoli, and spinach. It is important to note that vitamin C is water-soluble and not stored in the body, so regular intake is necessary.

- Vitamin D:

Vitamin D is another nutrient that plays a vital role in immune system function. It helps regulate the immune response and supports the activity of immune cells. Vitamin D also enhances the production of antimicrobial peptides, which are natural substances that help fight off infections.

Our bodies can produce vitamin D when our skin is exposed to sunlight. However, many people do not get enough sun exposure or have limited sun exposure due to lifestyle or geographical reasons. In such cases, dietary sources of vitamin D become important. Good food sources of vitamin D include fatty fish (such as salmon and mackerel), fortified dairy products, eggs, and mushrooms. Vitamin D supplements may also be necessary for individuals with low levels or those who have limited sun exposure.

- Zinc:

Zinc is an essential mineral that is involved in numerous immune system functions. It supports the development and function of immune cells, including white blood cells and natural killer cells. Zinc also helps regulate the inflammatory response and plays a role in wound healing.

Good food sources of zinc include oysters, beef, poultry, beans, nuts, and whole grains. Zinc supplements may be beneficial for individuals with zinc deficiency or those who have increased zinc requirements due to certain health conditions.

- Selenium:

Selenium is a trace mineral that acts as an antioxidant and supports immune system function. It helps regulate the production and activity of immune cells and enhances the body's response to infections. Selenium also plays a role in reducing inflammation and protecting against oxidative stress.

Good food sources of selenium include Brazil nuts, seafood (such as tuna and shrimp), eggs, and whole grains. Selenium supplements may be necessary for individuals with low selenium levels or those who have limited dietary intake.

- Vitamin A:

Vitamin A is essential for maintaining the integrity of the skin and mucous membranes, which act as barriers against pathogens. It also supports the production and function of white blood cells and enhances the immune response.

Good food sources of vitamin A include liver, fish, dairy products, eggs, carrots, sweet potatoes, and spinach. It is important to note that excessive intake of vitamin A can be toxic, so it is best to obtain it from food sources rather than supplements unless advised by a healthcare professional.

- Vitamin E:

Vitamin E is a powerful antioxidant that helps protect immune cells from oxidative damage. It also enhances the activity of immune cells and supports their function.

Good food sources of vitamin E include nuts (such as almonds and sunflower seeds), seeds, vegetable oils (such as sunflower oil), and spinach.

- Omega-3 fatty acids:

Omega-3 fatty acids are essential fats that play a crucial role in immune system function. They help regulate inflammation and support the activity of immune cells. Omega-3 fatty acids also enhance the production of anti-inflammatory molecules, which can help reduce the risk of chronic diseases.

Good food sources of omega-3 fatty acids include fatty fish (such as salmon and sardines), flaxseeds, chia seeds, and walnuts. Omega-3 fatty acid supplements, such as fish oil capsules, may be beneficial for individuals who do not consume enough dietary sources.

8. Probiotics:

Probiotics are beneficial bacteria that support a healthy gut microbiome. They help maintain a balanced immune response and enhance the function of immune cells. Probiotics also help prevent harmful bacteria from colonizing the gut and causing infections.

Good food sources of probiotics include yogurt, kefir, sauerkraut, kimchi, and other fermented foods. Probiotic supplements may be necessary for individuals with imbalances in their gut microbiome or those who have specific health conditions.

9. Iron:

Iron is an essential mineral that plays a vital role in immune system function. It is necessary for the production and maturation of immune cells, including white blood cells. Iron also supports the activity of immune cells and enhances their ability to fight off infections.

Good food sources of iron include lean meats, poultry, fish, beans, lentils, spinach, and fortified cereals. Iron supplements may be necessary for individuals with iron deficiency or those who have increased iron requirements due to certain health conditions.

10. B vitamins:

B vitamins, including B6, B9 (folate), and B12, are important for immune system function. They support the production and activity of immune cells and enhance the body's response to infections. B vitamins also play a role in energy production and help reduce fatigue.

Good food sources of B vitamins include whole grains, beans, lentils, leafy greens, poultry, fish, and eggs. B vitamin supplements may be necessary for individuals with deficiencies or those who have increased requirements.

It is important to note that while these essential nutrients play a crucial role in immune system support, they should not be considered a cure or treatment for specific diseases or infections. They are part of a holistic approach to maintaining good health and supporting immune function. It is always best to obtain these nutrients from whole foods as part of a well-balanced diet. However, in certain cases, dietary supplements may be necessary to fill in nutritional gaps. It is recommended to consult with a healthcare professional before starting any supplementation regimen, especially if you have underlying health conditions or are taking medications.

Chapter Three

Designing Your Disease-Fighting Diet

•*Creating a Balanced and Nutrient-Rich Eating Plan*

In a world where dietary trends, conflicting information, and a plethora of food choices abound, crafting a balanced and nutrient-rich eating plan can be both empowering and essential for optimal health. The foods we consume serve as the foundation for our well-being, influencing our energy levels, immune function, cognitive abilities, and overall vitality. A well-structured eating plan not only supports physical health but also fosters a positive relationship with food and nourishes the mind. This comprehensive guide delves into the principles and practices of creating a balanced and nutrient-rich eating plan that aligns with your individual needs, preferences, and goals.

Understanding the Basics: Macronutrients and Micronutrients

At the core of a balanced and nutrient-rich eating plan lie macronutrients and micronutrients, each playing a distinct yet interdependent role in maintaining health and supporting bodies micronutrient.

Macronutrients include carbohydrates, proteins, and fats. Carbohydrates provide the body with energy and are found in foods such as grains, fruits, vegetables, and legumes. They are divided into simple carbohydrates, which offer quick bursts of energy, and complex carbohydrates, which release energy gradually, promoting sustained fullness and stable blood sugar levels.

Proteins are the building blocks of life, essential for the growth, repair, and maintenance of tissues. They can be sourced from animal products like lean meats, poultry, fish, and dairy, as well as plant-based options like beans, lentils, and tofu. Incorporating a variety of protein sources ensures a diverse range of amino acids, supporting optimal bodily function.

Fats, once vilified, are essential for health when chosen wisely. Healthy fats, such as monounsaturated and polyunsaturated fats found in avocados, nuts, seeds, and fatty fish, play a crucial role in brain health, hormone production, and absorption of fat-soluble vitamins. Saturated fats and trans fats, often found in processed foods, should be consumed in moderation.

Micronutrients encompass vitamins and minerals, vital for various physiological processes. Vitamins like A, C, and E act as antioxidants, protecting cells from oxidative stress and bolstering immune function. Minerals like calcium, magnesium, and iron support bone health, muscle function, and oxygen transport. A diverse diet rich in fruits, vegetables, whole grains, lean proteins, and healthy fats ensures an array of micronutrients to fuel your body.

Why is a Balanced and Nutrient-Rich Eating Plan Important?

A balanced and nutrient-rich eating plan is important for several reasons:

1. Provides Essential Nutrients: A balanced eating plan ensures that you consume a variety of foods from different food groups, which helps provide your body with essential nutrients. These nutrients are necessary for proper growth, development, and maintenance of bodily functions.
2. Supports Optimal Health: A nutrient-rich eating plan supports overall health and reduces the risk of chronic diseases, such as heart disease, diabetes, and certain types of cancer. Consuming a wide range of nutrients helps maintain a healthy weight, supports cardiovascular health, strengthens the immune system, and promotes mental well-being.
3. Enhances Energy Levels: Proper nutrition is vital for energy production. A balanced eating plan provides the necessary macronutrients (carbohydrates, proteins, and fats) and micronutrients (vitamins and minerals) needed for optimal energy levels throughout the day.
4. Supports Weight Management: A balanced eating plan helps maintain a healthy weight by providing the body with the right balance of nutrients while controlling portion sizes. It

emphasizes whole, nutrient-dense foods that are lower in calories and higher in fiber, which can help promote satiety and prevent overeating.

5. Improves Digestive Health: A balanced eating plan includes foods rich in fiber, which helps support digestive health. Fiber adds bulk to the diet, promotes regular bowel movements, and supports the growth of beneficial gut bacteria. This can reduce the risk of constipation, promote a healthy gut microbiome, and support overall digestive health.

The Art of Balance: Creating a Nutrient-Dense Plate

A balanced and nutrient-rich eating plan involves more than just individual nutrients – it's about achieving harmony among various components on your plate. The "plate method" serves as a practical tool for constructing balanced meals.

Divide your plate into sections:

1. Fill half with colorful, non-starchy vegetables like leafy greens, bell peppers, and broccoli. These provide essential vitamins, minerals, and fiber.
2. Allocate a quarter for lean proteins such as grilled chicken, fish, tofu, or legumes. Proteins promote satiety, muscle maintenance, and immune function.
3. Dedicate the remaining quarter to whole grains or starchy vegetables like quinoa, brown rice, or sweet potatoes. Complex carbohydrates provide sustained energy and fiber.
4. Incorporate a source of healthy fat, such as olive oil, nuts, or seeds, to enhance flavor and aid nutrient absorption.

Mindful Eating: Savoring the Experience

Mindful eating goes beyond the physical act of consuming food – it involves being present and attentive to your eating experience. This practice fosters a deeper connection with your body's hunger and fullness cues, prevents overeating, and promotes a healthier relationship with food.

1. Engage your senses: Take time to appreciate the colors, textures, and aromas of your meal. Savor each bite, paying attention to the flavors and sensations in your mouth.
2. Eat with intention: Prioritize eating without distractions. Turn off screens, put away electronic devices, and create a peaceful environment that allows you to focus solely on your meal.
3. Listen to your body: Tune into your body's hunger and fullness signals. Eat when you're physically hungry and stop when you're comfortably satisfied, rather than when your plate is empty.

Practice gratitude: Cultivate an attitude of gratitude for the nourishment your meal provides. Acknowledge the effort that went into producing and preparing your food.

Flexibility and Variety: Nourishing Your Unique Needs

The beauty of a balanced and nutrient-rich eating plan lies in its flexibility and adaptability. There is no one-size-fits-all approach; rather, the goal is to create a plan that aligns with your individual needs, preferences, and lifestyle.

1. Embrace dietary variety: Incorporate a wide range of foods to ensure a diverse nutrient intake. Experiment with different fruits, vegetables, proteins, and grains to keep your meals exciting and satisfying.
2. Consider cultural and personal preferences: Your eating plan should reflect your cultural background, traditions, and personal tastes. Celebrate your heritage by incorporating traditional dishes that align with your nutritional goals.
3. Prioritize whole foods: Opt for minimally processed foods that retain their natural nutrients and flavors. Whole grains, fresh produce, lean proteins, and healthy fats should form the foundation of your eating plan.

Moderation, Not Deprivation: Enjoying Treats

A balanced and nutrient-rich eating plan recognizes the importance of indulging in treats occasionally. Restrictive diets often lead to cravings and unsustainable habits. Instead, practice moderation by enjoying your favorite treats mindfully and without guilt.

1. Practice the 80/20 rule: Strive to make 80% of your food choices nutrient-dense and aligned with your health goals. Allow yourself the flexibility to enjoy less nutrient-dense foods in moderation, making up the remaining 20%.

2. Listen to your cravings: If you're craving a particular treat, honor that craving rather than suppressing it. Savor the experience fully, and move on without dwelling on guilt.
3. Plan for social occasions: Special occasions and social gatherings often involve indulgent foods. Instead of avoiding such events, plan for them by making healthier choices leading up to the occasion.

Seek Professional Guidance: Working with Experts

Crafting a balanced and nutrient-rich eating plan can be overwhelming, especially when navigating complex dietary considerations. Seeking guidance from registered dietitians or nutritionists can provide personalized insights and support tailored to your unique needs.

1. Consultation and assessment: A registered dietitian or nutritionist will evaluate your current eating habits, lifestyle, and health goals to develop a customized eating plan that aligns with your objectives.
2. Education and empowerment: These professionals offer education on nutrition, portion control, and label reading, empowering you to make informed choices that support your well-being.
3. Nutritional strategies: Whether you're managing a medical condition, aiming for weight loss, or seeking performance optimization, a dietitian can offer evidence-based strategies to meet your goals.

Long-Term Sustainability: Building Lasting Habits

A balanced and nutrient-rich eating plan is not a short-term endeavor; it's a lifelong journey toward optimal health and vitality. Building sustainable habits requires patience, consistency, and a positive mindset.

1. Set realistic goals: Define achievable goals that are specific, measurable, and time-bound. Celebrate your progress along the way, regardless of how small it may seem.
2. Focus on progress, not perfection: Strive for improvement rather than perfection. Remember that setbacks are a natural part of the journey and offer opportunities for growth.
3. Cultivate a positive relationship with food: Shift your perspective from viewing food as mere fuel to appreciating it as a source of nourishment, pleasure, and social connection.

Reflect and adjust: Regularly assess your eating plan and habits. If something isn't working for you, don't hesitate to adjust your approach. Flexibility and adaptability are key to long-term success.

Tips for Creating a Balanced and Nutrient-Rich Eating Plan:

1. Include a Variety of Foods:

To ensure you get a wide range of nutrients, aim to include foods from all food groups in your eating plan. This includes:

- Fruits and vegetables: Aim for a variety of colorful fruits and vegetables, as they provide a wide range of vitamins, minerals, and antioxidants. Include both raw and cooked options to maximize nutrient intake.

- Whole grains: Choose whole grains, such as brown rice, quinoa, oats, and whole wheat bread, over refined grains. Whole grains are higher in fiber and provide more nutrients compared to refined grains.
- Lean proteins: Include lean sources of protein in your eating plan, such as poultry, fish, tofu, beans, lentils, and low-fat dairy products. Protein is essential for muscle growth and repair, as well as immune system function.
- Healthy fats: Incorporate sources of healthy fats into your eating plan, such as avocados, nuts, seeds, olive oil, and fatty fish. These fats provide essential fatty acids and support brain health.

2. Prioritize Nutrient-Dense Foods:

Focus on consuming nutrient-dense foods that provide a high amount of nutrients relative to their calorie content. These foods include fruits, vegetables, whole grains, lean proteins, and healthy fats. Nutrient-dense foods are rich in vitamins, minerals, fiber, and antioxidants, which are essential for optimal health.

3. Control Portion Sizes:

While it is important to include a variety of foods in your eating plan, portion control is key to maintaining a healthy weight. Be mindful of portion sizes and listen to your body's hunger and fullness cues. Use smaller plates and bowls to help control portion sizes visually.

4. Limit Processed and Sugary Foods:

Processed and sugary foods are often high in calories, unhealthy fats, added sugars, and sodium, while being low in nutrients. Limit your intake of these foods, including sugary beverages, processed snacks, fast food, and desserts. Instead, opt for whole, unprocessed foods whenever possible.

5. Hydrate Properly:

Proper hydration is essential for overall health and well-being. Aim to drink an adequate amount of water throughout the day to stay hydrated. Limit your intake of sugary beverages and opt for water, herbal tea, or infused water instead.

6. Practice Mindful Eating:

Practice mindful eating by paying attention to your body's hunger and fullness cues. Eat slowly, savor each bite, and listen to your body's signals of satiety. This can help prevent overeating and promote a healthier relationship with food.

7. Plan and Prepare Meals:

Planning and preparing meals in advance can help ensure that you have nutritious options readily available. Set aside time each week to plan your meals, create a grocery list, and prepare meals in advance. This can help you make healthier choices and avoid relying on unhealthy convenience foods.

8. Seek Professional Guidance:

If you are unsure about how to create a balanced and nutrient-rich eating plan, consider seeking guidance from a registered dietitian or nutritionist. They can provide personalized recommendations based on your specific needs, preferences, and health goals.

In conclusion, creating a balanced and nutrient-rich eating plan is crucial for supporting overall health and well-being. It provides the body with essential nutrients, supports optimal immune system function, enhances energy levels, promotes weight management, and improves digestive health. By incorporating a variety of foods from different food groups, prioritizing nutrient-dense options, controlling portion sizes, and practicing mindful eating, you can create a sustainable eating plan that supports your health goals. Remember to seek professional guidance if needed and make gradual changes for long-term success.

•*Tailoring Your Diet to Specific Health Goals*

The foods we consume play a profound role in shaping our health and well-being. In the intricate dance between diet and health, the notion of "one-size-fits-all" no longer suffices. Tailoring your diet to specific health goals has gained prominence as individuals recognize the potential of personalized nutrition to optimize their physical, mental, and emotional health. Whether you're aiming for weight loss, managing a medical condition, enhancing athletic performance, or cultivating overall wellness, understanding how to customize your diet to align with your unique objectives is a powerful tool on your journey to better health.

Defining Your Health Goals: The First Step

Before embarking on any dietary changes, it's essential to define your health goals with clarity. Your objectives could range from weight management, improved cardiovascular health, better blood sugar control, increased energy levels, enhanced athletic performance, or simply feeling more vibrant and balanced. Setting specific, measurable, achievable, relevant, and time-bound (SMART) goals lays the foundation for a focused and effective approach.

For instance, if your goal is weight loss, determine the amount of weight you want to lose and the timeframe in which you aim to achieve it. If you're focused on managing diabetes, establish target blood sugar levels and understand how dietary modifications can contribute to achieving those targets.

Weight loss

If weight loss is your primary goal, there are several key principles to keep in mind when tailoring your diet:

1. Create a Calorie Deficit: To lose weight, you need to consume fewer calories than you burn. Start by calculating your daily calorie needs and aim for a moderate calorie deficit of around 500-1000 calories per day. This will result in a gradual and sustainable weight loss of 1-2 pounds per week.

2. Focus on Nutrient Density: While reducing calories is important for weight loss, it's equally crucial to prioritize nutrient-dense foods. These are foods that are low in calories but high in vitamins, minerals, and other beneficial compounds. Fill your plate with fruits, vegetables, whole grains, lean proteins, and healthy fats to ensure you're getting the nutrients your body needs while still creating a calorie deficit.

3. Watch Portion Sizes: Even if you're eating healthy foods, consuming too much of them can hinder weight loss. Be mindful of portion sizes and practice portion control. Use smaller plates and bowls, measure out serving sizes, and listen to your body's hunger and fullness cues.

4. Monitor Macronutrient Balance: While there is no one-size-fits-all approach to macronutrient balance for weight loss, many people find success with a balanced approach that includes a moderate intake of carbohydrates, proteins, and fats. Experiment with different ratios to see what works best for you and consult with a registered dietitian if needed.

Muscle Gain

If your goal is to build muscle, your diet should focus on providing the nutrients necessary for muscle growth and repair. Consider the following tips:

1. Increase Protein Intake: Protein is the building block of muscles, so it's essential to consume enough to support muscle growth. Aim for 1.2-2 grams of protein per kilogram of body weight per day, depending on your activity level and goals. Include lean sources of protein such as chicken, turkey, fish, tofu, beans, lentils, and low-fat dairy products in each meal.

2. Eat Sufficient Calories: To build muscle, you need to consume enough calories to support the energy demands of your workouts and provide the building blocks for muscle growth. Calculate your daily calorie needs and aim for a slight calorie surplus of around 250-500 calories per day.

3. Prioritize Strength Training: In addition to proper nutrition, strength training is crucial for building muscle. Focus on compound exercises that target multiple muscle groups, such as squats, deadlifts, bench presses, and rows. Aim to progressively overload your muscles by gradually increasing the weight or intensity of your workouts over time.

4. Time Your Nutrition: To optimize muscle growth, it's important to fuel your body before and after workouts. Consume a pre-workout snack or meal that includes carbohydrates for energy and protein for muscle repair. After your workout, consume a post-workout meal or snack that includes protein and carbohydrates to replenish glycogen stores and support muscle recovery.

Managing Health Conditions

If you're managing a specific health condition, such as diabetes, high blood pressure, or gastrointestinal issues, tailoring your diet is crucial for supporting your health. Consider the following tips:

1. Consult with a Healthcare Professional: If you have a specific health condition, it's important to work closely with a healthcare professional, such as a registered dietitian or doctor, to develop a tailored eating plan. They can provide personalized recommendations based on your specific condition, medications, and individual needs.
2. Focus on Whole, Unprocessed Foods: Regardless of the specific health condition you're managing, prioritizing whole, unprocessed foods is essential. These foods are rich in nutrients and fiber and can help support overall health. Aim to include a variety of fruits, vegetables, whole grains, lean proteins, and healthy fats in your diet.
3. Monitor Carbohydrate Intake: For conditions such as diabetes or insulin resistance, monitoring carbohydrate intake is important for managing blood sugar levels. Work with a healthcare professional to determine the appropriate amount and type of carbohydrates for your specific needs. Consider choosing complex carbohydrates that are high in fiber and have a lower impact on blood sugar levels.
4. Reduce Sodium Intake: If you have high blood pressure or other cardiovascular conditions, reducing sodium intake can be beneficial. Limit your consumption of processed foods, which are often high in sodium, and opt for fresh, homemade meals instead. Use herbs, spices, and other flavorings to enhance the taste of your food without relying on salt.

Enhancing Athletic Performance

If you're an athlete or someone who engages in regular physical activity, tailoring your diet to support performance and recovery is crucial. Consider the following tips:

1. Prioritize Carbohydrates: Carbohydrates are the primary fuel source for physical activity, so it's important to consume enough to support your energy needs. Aim for a diet that includes a variety of complex carbohydrates, such as whole grains, fruits, vegetables, and legumes. Consider timing your carbohydrate intake around workouts to optimize performance and recovery.
2. Include Adequate Protein: Protein is important for muscle repair and recovery, so make sure you're consuming enough to support your activity level. Aim for 1.2-2 grams of protein per kilogram of body weight per day, depending on the intensity and duration of your workouts. Include lean sources of protein in each meal and snack, such as chicken, turkey, fish, tofu, beans, lentils, and low-fat dairy products.
3. Stay Hydrated: Proper hydration is crucial for athletic performance and recovery. Aim to drink an adequate amount of water throughout the day and increase your fluid intake during workouts or intense physical activity. Consider weighing yourself before and after exercise to estimate fluid losses and drink enough to replace those losses.
4. Consider Sports-Specific Supplements: Depending on your specific sport or activity, you may benefit from certain sports supplements. Consult with a registered dietitian or sports nutritionist to determine if supplements such as creatine, beta-alanine, or caffeine may be appropriate for your goals and individual needs.

Consulting a Healthcare Professional: Expert Guidance

Once your health goals are clearly defined, consulting a healthcare professional can provide invaluable guidance. A registered dietitian, nutritionist, or medical doctor with expertise in nutrition can help translate your goals into a practical and evidence-based dietary plan. These professionals consider your individual health status, medical history, dietary preferences, and lifestyle when crafting recommendations tailored to your needs.

A registered dietitian, in particular, can assess your dietary intake, identify areas for improvement, and create a personalized eating plan that optimally supports your health objectives. Whether you're managing chronic conditions like heart disease, diabetes, or gastrointestinal issues, or aiming to enhance athletic performance, their expertise can help you navigate dietary complexities and implement sustainable changes.

Caloric Needs and Macros: A Foundation for Customization

Understanding your caloric needs and macronutrient distribution forms the basis for tailoring your diet to your health goals. Macronutrients – carbohydrates, proteins, and fats – provide energy and fulfill essential bodily functions. The proportions in which you consume these macronutrients can be adjusted based on your objectives.

For instance, weight loss often involves creating a calorie deficit, where you consume fewer calories than you expend. This typically involves reducing your carbohydrate intake while ensuring adequate protein and healthy fat consumption to preserve muscle mass and support satiety. On the other hand, athletes seeking to optimize performance may require higher carbohydrate intake to fuel workouts and replenish glycogen stores.

Micros for Health: Meeting Nutrient Needs

In addition to macronutrients, micronutrients – vitamins and minerals – are critical for overall health. Tailoring your diet to specific health goals involves ensuring you meet your nutrient requirements.

For example, if you're pursuing a plant-based diet, paying attention to vitamin B12 intake is crucial, as this vitamin is primarily found in animal products. If you're aiming to enhance bone health, ensuring adequate calcium and vitamin D intake is paramount. Micronutrient-rich foods like colorful fruits and vegetables, whole grains, lean proteins, and healthy fats should form the basis of your diet to provide a wide array of essential nutrients.

Mind-Body Connection: Nurturing Mental Health

Dietary choices don't solely influence physical health; they also impact mental well-being. Tailoring your diet to support mental health involves consuming nutrients that promote brain health and mood stability.

Omega-3 fatty acids, found in fatty fish, flaxseeds, and walnuts, are associated with cognitive function and mood regulation. B vitamins, particularly folate and B12, play a role in neurotransmitter synthesis and may impact mood. Antioxidant-rich foods like berries, leafy greens, and nuts protect against oxidative stress, which can contribute to mental health disorders.

Cultivating a Diet That Supports Longevity: Anti-Inflammatory Approach

An anti-inflammatory eating plan is gaining attention for its potential to support longevity and reduce the risk of chronic diseases. Tailoring your diet to an anti-inflammatory approach involves emphasizing foods that reduce inflammation and oxidative stress.

Anti-inflammatory foods include colorful fruits and vegetables, fatty fish rich in omega-3s, nuts, seeds, olive oil, and spices like turmeric. Reducing the consumption of processed foods, refined sugars, and trans fats can also contribute to an anti-inflammatory eating pattern.

The Role of Mindfulness: Honoring Your Body

As you tailor your diet to your health goals, mindfulness serves as a powerful companion. Mindful eating involves being present during meals, savoring each bite, and listening to your body's hunger and fullness cues.

Practice mindful eating by:

- Eating without distractions, such as phones or screens.
- Paying attention to the flavors, textures, and aromas of your food.
- Eating slowly and savoring each bite.
- Recognizing the difference between true hunger and emotional triggers.

Adapting Over Time: A Lifelong Journey

Health goals evolve over time, and your dietary approach should adapt accordingly. Regularly assessing your progress, revisiting your goals, and seeking guidance from healthcare professionals ensures that your eating plan remains aligned with your current needs.

Practical Tips for Success

Regardless of your specific health goals, there are several practical tips that can help you succeed in tailoring your diet:

1. Set Realistic and Specific Goals: Set realistic and specific goals that are measurable and achievable. Instead of saying "I want to lose weight," set a specific target, such as "I want to lose 10 pounds in three months." This will help you stay focused and motivated.
2. Keep a Food Diary: Keeping a food diary can help you become more aware of your eating habits and identify areas for improvement. Write down everything you eat and drink, including portion sizes and any symptoms or reactions you may experience. This can help you identify patterns and make necessary adjustments.
3. Meal Prep and Planning: Plan your meals in advance and prepare them in bulk if possible. This can help save time and ensure that you have nutritious options readily available. Set aside time each week to plan your meals, create a grocery list, and prepare meals in advance.
4. Seek Support: Don't be afraid to seek support from friends, family, or professionals. Share your goals with others and ask for their support and encouragement. Consider joining a support group or working with a registered dietitian or nutritionist who can provide guidance and accountability.
5. Practice Mindful Eating: Practice mindful eating by paying attention to your body's hunger and fullness cues. Eat slowly, savor each bite, and listen to your body's signals of satiety. This can help prevent overeating and promote a healthier relationship with food.

6. Be Flexible: Remember that nutrition is not an all-or-nothing approach. It's okay to indulge in your favorite treats occasionally or deviate from your plan from time to time. The key is to practice moderation and make sustainable choices that align with your goals in the long run.

Tailoring your diet to specific health goals is a dynamic process that involves understanding your objectives, seeking expert guidance, adjusting macronutrient ratios, meeting micronutrient needs, and considering the interplay of diet and health conditions. Whether you're pursuing weight management, managing chronic conditions, enhancing athletic performance, nurturing mental health, or promoting longevity, a personalized approach to nutrition empowers you to make choices that optimize your well-being. Remember, your dietary journey is unique and ongoing – a reflection of your commitment to health and self-care.

Chapter Four

Foods that Combat Common Ailments

•*Heart-Healthy Diet Choices and Cardiovascular Disease Prevention*

The heart, a tireless worker, sustains life by pumping blood throughout the body. As the central organ of our circulatory system, its health is paramount for overall well-being. Cardiovascular diseases (CVDs), including heart disease and stroke, continue to be leading causes of morbidity and mortality worldwide. The good news is that many risk factors for CVDs, such as unhealthy dietary habits, are modifiable. Adopting a heart-healthy diet can significantly reduce the risk of developing these conditions. This comprehensive guide explores the principles and practices of making diet choices that promote heart health and contribute to the prevention of cardiovascular diseases.

Understanding Cardiovascular Diseases: The Role of Diet

Cardiovascular diseases encompass a range of conditions affecting the heart and blood vessels, including coronary artery disease, heart failure, and stroke. These conditions often share common risk factors, and many are linked to lifestyle choices, particularly diet.

A heart-healthy diet plays a pivotal role in preventing and managing CVDs by addressing risk factors such as high blood pressure, high cholesterol levels, obesity, and inflammation. Adopting dietary habits that support heart health not only reduces the likelihood of developing CVDs but also contributes to overall well-being.

Key Principles of a Heart-Healthy Diet

1. Prioritize Fruits and Vegetables: A cornerstone of a heart-healthy diet is the consumption of a variety of colorful fruits and vegetables. These nutrient-rich foods provide vitamins, minerals, antioxidants, and dietary fiber that promote heart health. Aim to fill half your plate with fruits and vegetables at each meal.
2. Choose Whole Grains: Whole grains like brown rice, quinoa, whole wheat, and oats are rich in fiber and nutrients that help regulate blood sugar levels and maintain healthy cholesterol levels. Opt for whole grains over refined grains to support heart health.

3. Opt for Lean Proteins: Choose lean sources of protein such as poultry, fish, beans, legumes, and tofu. These options are lower in saturated fat and cholesterol, reducing the risk of heart disease. Fatty fish, like salmon and mackerel, are particularly beneficial due to their omega-3 fatty acids, which promote heart health.

4. Embrace Healthy Fats: Not all fats are created equal. Replace saturated and trans fats with heart-healthy unsaturated fats like those found in olive oil, avocados, nuts, and seeds. These fats can help lower bad cholesterol levels and reduce inflammation.

5. Limit Sodium Intake: Excessive salt intake can contribute to high blood pressure, a major risk factor for heart disease. Opt for fresh foods over processed ones, and use herbs and spices to add flavor to your meals without relying on salt.

6. Manage Portion Sizes: Portion control is key to maintaining a healthy weight and preventing overeating. Be mindful of portion sizes and listen to your body's hunger and fullness cues.

7. Reduce Added Sugars: High intake of added sugars has been linked to obesity, diabetes, and heart disease. Minimize sugary beverages, snacks, and desserts in favor of whole, natural foods.

8. Moderate Alcohol Consumption: If you choose to consume alcohol, do so in moderation. For men, this generally means up to two drinks per day, and for women, up to one drink per day. Red wine, in particular, has been associated with heart health due to its antioxidants.

9. Stay Hydrated: Water is essential for heart health, as it helps maintain blood volume and supports proper circulation. Aim to drink plenty of water throughout the day.

10. Practice Mindful Eating: Eating mindfully, paying attention to your food and how it makes you feel, can help prevent overeating and promote a healthier relationship with food.

Reducing Risk Factors Through Diet

1. Lowering Cholesterol Levels: High levels of low-density lipoprotein (LDL) cholesterol, often referred to as "bad" cholesterol, are associated with an increased risk of heart disease. Dietary strategies to lower LDL cholesterol include:

- Consuming soluble fiber found in oats, legumes, fruits, and vegetables.
- Replacing saturated fats with unsaturated fats from sources like olive oil, nuts, and fatty fish.
- Including plant sterols found in fortified foods like margarine.

2. Managing Blood Pressure: High blood pressure is a significant risk factor for heart disease. Dietary approaches to managing blood pressure include:

- Reducing sodium intake by avoiding processed and packaged foods high in salt.
- Consuming potassium-rich foods like bananas, spinach, and beans.
- Incorporating magnesium-rich foods like nuts, seeds, and whole grains.

3. Controlling Blood Sugar: Diabetes and uncontrolled blood sugar levels increase the risk of CVDs. Dietary strategies to manage blood sugar include:
- Choosing whole grains and fiber-rich foods to prevent rapid spikes in blood sugar.
- Monitoring carbohydrate intake and spreading it evenly throughout the day.

- Opting for lean proteins to help stabilize blood sugar levels.

4. Reducing Inflammation: Chronic inflammation is associated with the development of CVDs. Anti-inflammatory dietary choices include:
- Incorporating fatty fish rich in omega-3 fatty acids.
- Consuming antioxidant-rich foods like berries, leafy greens, and nuts.
- Minimizing consumption of processed and fried foods.

Lifestyle and Behavioral Factors

While a heart-healthy diet is a cornerstone of cardiovascular disease prevention, it's important to remember that dietary choices are just one piece of the puzzle. Other lifestyle factors play a significant role in promoting heart health:

1. Regular Physical Activity: Engaging in regular exercise supports heart health by improving cardiovascular fitness, maintaining a healthy weight, and reducing risk factors like high blood pressure and high cholesterol levels.
2. Stress Management: Chronic stress can contribute to heart disease. Practicing stress-reduction techniques such as meditation, deep breathing, yoga, and spending time in nature can support heart health.
3. Adequate Sleep: Poor sleep patterns are associated with an increased risk of heart disease. Prioritize quality sleep by maintaining a regular sleep schedule and creating a sleep-conducive environment.
4. Tobacco Cessation: Smoking is a major risk factor for heart disease. Quitting smoking is one of the most significant steps you can take to improve heart health.
5. Regular Health Check-ups: Regular medical check-ups allow for the monitoring of risk factors like blood pressure, cholesterol levels, and blood sugar. Work with your healthcare provider to develop a comprehensive plan for heart health.

Promoting heart health through diet is an empowering journey that involves making mindful choices, embracing nutrient-rich foods, and adopting a lifestyle that supports overall well-being. By understanding the principles of a heart-healthy diet, reducing risk factors, and

Incorporating heart-protective behaviors, you can significantly reduce the risk of cardiovascular diseases and enjoy a life marked by vitality and longevity. Remember, each meal is an opportunity to nourish your heart and invest in your health.

•Anti-Inflammatory Foods for Joint Health and Pain Management

Joint health is integral to our overall mobility, allowing us to perform daily activities with ease and comfort. However, as we age or face certain health conditions, joint pain and inflammation can become unwelcome companions. Chronic joint pain, often caused by conditions like osteoarthritis or rheumatoid arthritis, can significantly impact our quality of life. While medications and medical interventions play a role in managing joint pain, the potential of incorporating anti-inflammatory foods into our diet is gaining recognition. This comprehensive guide explores the science behind anti-inflammatory foods, their impact on joint health, and their role in managing pain.

Understanding Inflammation: The Culprit Behind Joint Pain

Inflammation is a fundamental biological response designed to protect the body from harm. It's the immune system's natural defense mechanism against infections, injuries, and toxins. In its acute form, inflammation is a short-lived and necessary process that promotes healing and tissue repair. However, when inflammation becomes chronic or excessive, it can lead to a host of health issues, including joint pain.

Imagine you accidentally cut your finger while preparing a meal. Within moments, you might notice the area becoming red, warm, and swollen. This is a classic example of acute inflammation in action. The immune system rushes immune cells, white blood cells, and healing molecules to the injured site to initiate repairs. The increased blood flow results in the familiar signs of redness and warmth, while swelling occurs due to the accumulation of fluids and immune cells that help to fight off potential infections.

Once the healing process is complete, the acute inflammation subsides, and the injured area returns to normal. This type of inflammation is a vital response that allows your body to repair damage efficiently.

While acute inflammation is essential for maintaining health, chronic inflammation is a different story. Chronic inflammation occurs when the body's inflammatory response persists over an extended period, often due to ongoing triggers such as poor diet, lack of exercise, smoking, excessive stress, or certain medical conditions.

Inflammation, in its chronic form, becomes a double-edged sword. It can contribute to the development of various diseases, including cardiovascular disease, diabetes, and even cancer. In particular, chronic inflammation plays a significant role in joint pain and diseases like osteoarthritis and rheumatoid arthritis.

Osteoarthritis (OA) is the most common form of arthritis, affecting millions of people worldwide. It primarily involves the degeneration of joint cartilage, the tissue that cushions the

ends of bones within a joint. As cartilage breaks down, bones can start to rub against each other, causing pain, stiffness, and reduced mobility.

Chronic inflammation is a key player in the development and progression of OA. In response to the ongoing degradation of cartilage, the body's immune system releases inflammatory molecules, including cytokines, that contribute to further tissue damage. This creates a vicious cycle where inflammation perpetuates cartilage breakdown and worsens joint pain.

Rheumatoid arthritis (RA) is an autoimmune disease characterized by inflammation in multiple joints. Unlike OA, where the primary problem is cartilage breakdown, RA involves the immune system attacking healthy joint tissues.

In RA, the immune system mistakenly identifies joint tissues as foreign invaders and launches an immune response against them. This results in chronic inflammation within the joints, leading to pain, swelling, and joint damage over time.

Inflammation in RA is particularly destructive because it doesn't only target the cartilage but also affects the synovium, the tissue lining the joint capsule. The inflamed synovium can erode cartilage, damage bone, and even cause joint deformities.

As the common denominator in joint pain conditions like OA and RA, inflammation becomes a central focus in pain management strategies. While medications and medical interventions play crucial roles, lifestyle choices, including dietary habits, are gaining recognition for their potential to mitigate inflammation and support joint health.

The Role of Diet in Inflammation and Joint Health

Diet plays a significant role in inflammation and joint health. Certain foods can either promote or reduce inflammation in the body, which can directly impact joint pain and overall joint health.

Inflammation is a natural response by the immune system to protect the body from injury or infection. However, chronic inflammation can lead to various health conditions, including joint pain and arthritis. A diet high in processed foods, refined sugars, unhealthy fats, and excessive alcohol consumption can contribute to chronic inflammation.

On the other hand, an anti-inflammatory diet can help reduce inflammation and support joint health. This type of diet typically includes foods that are rich in antioxidants, omega-3 fatty acids, and phytochemicals. These nutrients have been shown to have anti-inflammatory properties and can help reduce joint pain.

Fruits and vegetables are an essential part of an anti-inflammatory diet as they are rich in antioxidants and phytochemicals. Berries, leafy greens, and cruciferous vegetables are particularly beneficial due to their high antioxidant content. Whole grains, such as brown rice and quinoa, provide fiber and important nutrients that support overall health, including joint health.

Healthy fats, such as those found in fatty fish (salmon, mackerel), nuts, seeds, and olive oil, are also important for reducing inflammation. These foods contain omega-3 fatty acids, which have been shown to have anti-inflammatory effects. Omega-3 fatty acids can help reduce joint stiffness and pain associated with arthritis.

In addition to incorporating anti-inflammatory foods, it is important to avoid or limit foods that can promote inflammation. This includes processed foods, sugary beverages, refined carbohydrates, and unhealthy fats (trans fats and saturated fats). These foods can increase inflammation in the body and worsen joint pain.

It is worth noting that while diet can play a significant role in managing inflammation and joint pain, it is not a standalone solution. Other lifestyle factors, such as regular exercise, stress management, and adequate sleep, also contribute to overall joint health. Therefore, a comprehensive approach that includes dietary modifications alongside other lifestyle changes is crucial for managing joint pain and promoting joint health.

It is important to consult with a healthcare professional or registered dietitian to personalize the diet and ensure that it meets individual needs and preferences. They can provide guidance, support, and specific recommendations based on an individual's unique circumstances and health conditions.

Anti-Inflammatory Foods: Nourishing Your Joints

1. Fatty Fish: Fatty fish like salmon, mackerel, sardines, and trout are rich sources of omega-3 fatty acids, known for their anti-inflammatory properties. Omega-3s can help reduce inflammation and ease joint pain by inhibiting the production of inflammatory compounds.

2. Berries: Berries such as strawberries, blueberries, and cherries are packed with antioxidants called anthocyanins. These compounds have been shown to reduce inflammation and oxidative stress, potentially benefiting joint health.
3. Leafy Greens: Dark leafy greens like spinach, kale, and Swiss chard are abundant in vitamins, minerals, and antioxidants. They also contain phytonutrients with anti-inflammatory effects that can contribute to joint health.
4. Nuts and Seeds: Walnuts, almonds, flaxseeds, and chia seeds are rich in healthy fats, including omega-3s and monounsaturated fats. These fats have anti-inflammatory properties that can alleviate joint discomfort.
5. Turmeric and Ginger: Curcumin, the active compound in turmeric, and gingerol in ginger are known for their potent anti-inflammatory effects. Incorporating these spices into your diet can help manage joint pain.
6. Olive Oil: Extra-virgin olive oil is rich in monounsaturated fats and polyphenols that possess anti-inflammatory properties. It can be a healthy substitute for other cooking oils and dressings.
7. Beans and Legumes: Beans and legumes are excellent sources of plant-based protein, fiber, and antioxidants. They contribute to a balanced diet that supports joint health and may help manage inflammation.

8. Whole Grains: Whole grains like brown rice, quinoa, and whole wheat are high in fiber and nutrients. Their complex carbohydrates release energy slowly, preventing blood sugar spikes that can contribute to inflammation.
9. Spices: In addition to turmeric and ginger, other spices like cinnamon and garlic have been shown to possess anti-inflammatory and immune-modulating properties.
10. Green Tea: Green tea is rich in catechins, antioxidants that have been associated with reduced inflammation and improved joint health.

The Science Behind Anti-Inflammatory Foods

Several mechanisms underlie the anti-inflammatory effects of these foods:

1. Omega-3 fatty acids found in fatty fish and certain seeds inhibit the production of inflammatory molecules called prostaglandins and leukotrienes.
2. Antioxidants in berries, leafy greens, and other colorful fruits and vegetables neutralize free radicals that contribute to inflammation.
3. Phytonutrients like quercetin in apples, onions, and citrus fruits inhibit inflammatory enzymes.
4. Curcumin in turmeric and gingerol in ginger modulate the activity of inflammatory pathways.
5. Fiber-rich foods support gut health and influence the gut microbiome, which has a role in inflammation regulation.

Building a Joint-Friendly Eating Plan

Creating a diet that supports joint health involves more than individual foods; it's about adopting an overall eating pattern that prioritizes anti-inflammatory choices. Here's how to structure your meals:

1. Emphasize Fruits and Vegetables: Aim to fill half your plate with a colorful array of fruits and vegetables. These foods provide a diverse range of antioxidants and nutrients.
2. Choose Whole Grains: Opt for whole grains like quinoa, brown rice, and oats over refined grains. Whole grains offer more fiber and nutrients that support inflammation control.

3. Include Lean Proteins: Incorporate lean protein sources such as poultry, fish, beans, and legumes. Protein is essential for tissue repair and overall health.
4. Incorporate Healthy Fats: Include sources of healthy fats like fatty fish, nuts, seeds, and olive oil. These fats support joint health and contribute to an anti-inflammatory diet.
5. Spice Up Your Meals: Use herbs and spices like turmeric, ginger, garlic, and cinnamon to add flavor and anti-inflammatory benefits to your dishes.

6. Hydrate Wisely: Opt for water, herbal teas, and green tea as your main beverages. Limit sugary drinks and excessive caffeine, which can contribute to inflammation.
7. Limit Processed Foods: Minimize your consumption of processed foods, sugary snacks, and high-sodium meals, as these can exacerbate inflammation.
8. Practice Portion Control: Maintain appropriate portion sizes to prevent overeating, as excess weight can worsen joint pain.
9. Mindful Eating: Practice mindful eating by savoring each bite, chewing slowly, and paying attention to your body's hunger and fullness cues.
10. Stay Hydrated: Drink plenty of water throughout the day to support joint lubrication and overall hydration.

The Importance of Personalization

Personalization is crucial in anti-inflammatory foods and joint pain management because everyone's body is unique and may respond differently to certain foods and dietary approaches. Joint pain can be caused by various factors, including inflammation, arthritis, injury, or underlying health conditions. Therefore, it is important to tailor the diet to each individual's specific needs and preferences.

By personalizing the approach to anti-inflammatory foods and joint pain management, individuals can identify and eliminate potential trigger foods that may exacerbate inflammation and joint pain. This involves keeping a food diary and tracking symptoms to identify patterns and correlations between certain foods and flare-ups. For example, some individuals may find that consuming nightshade vegetables (such as tomatoes, peppers, and eggplants) worsens their joint pain, while others may not experience any negative effects.

Furthermore, personalization allows individuals to focus on foods that have been shown to have anti-inflammatory properties and promote joint health. While there are general guidelines for an anti-inflammatory diet (such as consuming plenty of fruits, vegetables, whole grains, and healthy fats), personalization allows for individual preferences and dietary restrictions. For instance, individuals who follow a plant-based or vegetarian diet can still incorporate anti-inflammatory foods such as legumes, nuts, seeds, and plant-based oils.

In addition to personalizing the food choices, it is also important to consider other lifestyle factors that can impact joint health, such as exercise, stress management, and adequate sleep. Personalization allows individuals to create a holistic approach to joint pain management that addresses their unique needs and circumstances.

Overall, personalization in anti-inflammatory foods and joint pain management is essential for optimizing outcomes and improving quality of life. By tailoring the diet to individual needs and preferences, individuals can identify trigger foods, incorporate anti-inflammatory foods, and create a comprehensive approach that addresses all aspects of joint health. Consulting with a

healthcare professional or registered dietitian can provide personalized guidance and support in managing joint pain through dietary modifications.

Lifestyle Factors for Joint Health

While anti-inflammatory foods play a significant role in managing joint pain, lifestyle factors also contribute to overall joint health:

1. Regular Physical Activity: Engage in low-impact exercises like swimming, walking, or cycling to strengthen muscles around the joints and improve flexibility.
2. Weight Management: Maintaining a healthy weight reduces the load on your joints and can alleviate joint pain.
3. Stress Management: Chronic stress can exacerbate inflammation. Incorporate stress-reduction techniques such as meditation, deep breathing, and yoga into your routine.
4. Ergonomic Practices: Maintain proper posture and use ergonomic tools to reduce strain on your joints during daily activities.
5. Rest and Recovery: Prioritize quality sleep and allow your body ample time to rest and recover between physical activities.
6. Medical Management: If you're experiencing chronic joint pain, consult a healthcare professional for a comprehensive evaluation and personalized treatment plan.

Incorporating anti-inflammatory foods into your diet is a proactive step toward supporting joint health and managing pain. By focusing on nutrient-rich foods, adopting an anti-inflammatory eating pattern, and considering individual needs, you can potentially reduce inflammation, improve joint function, and enhance your overall quality of life. Remember, dietary choices are just one aspect of a comprehensive approach to joint health – a journey that combines mindful eating, regular movement, and holistic well-being.

•Nutritional Strategies for Diabetes Management and Prevention

Diabetes, a chronic condition characterized by high blood sugar levels, affects millions of people worldwide. Its impact on overall health is substantial, and managing or preventing diabetes requires a multifaceted approach. Nutrition plays a pivotal role in diabetes management and prevention, offering a powerful tool for controlling blood sugar levels, reducing complications,

and improving quality of life. This comprehensive guide explores the science behind diabetes, the role of nutrition, and effective strategies for managing and preventing this condition.

Understanding Diabetes: Types and IImpac

Diabetes is divided into different types, each with its distinct characteristics:

1. Type 1 Diabetes: An autoimmune condition where the immune system attacks and destroys insulin-producing cells in the pancreas. People with type 1 diabetes rely on insulin injections to manage their blood sugar levels.
2. Type 2 Diabetes: The most common form of diabetes, often linked to obesity and sedentary lifestyles. In type 2 diabetes, cells become resistant to insulin's effects, leading to elevated blood sugar levels.
3. Gestational Diabetes: Occurs during pregnancy when the body can't produce enough insulin to meet the increased demands, leading to high blood sugar levels.
4. Prediabetes: A precursor to type 2 diabetes, where blood sugar levels are higher than normal but not high enough to be classified as diabetes. Prediabetes is a warning sign, indicating a higher risk of developing type 2 diabetes.

Uncontrolled diabetes can lead to severe complications, including cardiovascular disease, kidney damage, nerve damage, vision impairment, and poor wound healing. The goal of diabetes management and prevention is to keep blood sugar levels within a healthy range to minimize these risks.

The Role of Nutrition in Diabetes Management

Nutrition is a cornerstone of diabetes management because the foods we eat directly influence blood sugar levels. Effective nutritional strategies can help stabilize blood sugar, improve insulin sensitivity, and reduce the risk of complications. When crafting a diabetes-focused eating plan, several key principles come into play:

1. Carbohydrate Management: Carbohydrates have the most significant impact on blood sugar levels. Carbohydrates are broken down into glucose (sugar) during digestion, leading to an increase in blood sugar. Monitoring carbohydrate intake and choosing complex carbohydrates, which release glucose more gradually, can help stabilize blood sugar levels.
2. Glycemic Index (GI): The glycemic index categorizes carbohydrates based on how quickly they raise blood sugar levels. Low-GI foods have a slower and steadier impact on blood sugar, making them beneficial choices for diabetes management.
3. Portion Control: Managing portion sizes helps control calorie intake and blood sugar levels. Balancing carbohydrate, protein, and healthy fat portions contributes to more stable blood sugar throughout the day.

4. Protein and Fat: Including lean protein and healthy fats in meals can slow down the digestion of carbohydrates, preventing rapid spikes in blood sugar. Protein and fat also contribute to satiety and help manage appetite.
5. Fiber-Rich Foods: Fiber slows the absorption of glucose and helps maintain steady blood sugar levels. Incorporating whole grains, legumes, vegetables, and fruits into your diet provides ample fiber.
6. Sugar and Sweeteners: Minimizing added sugars and opting for natural sweeteners in moderation is crucial for diabetes management. Artificial sweeteners can be used as alternatives but should be consumed judiciously.
7. Hydration: Staying hydrated supports overall health and can help regulate blood sugar levels. Choose water, herbal teas, and other non-caloric beverages over sugary drinks.

Strategies for Diabetes Management and Prevention

1. Balanced Eating: Creating balanced meals that include a variety of nutrients helps manage blood sugar levels. Aim to include a source of protein, healthy fat, complex carbohydrates, and plenty of non-starchy vegetables in each meal.

2. Regular Monitoring: Regularly checking blood sugar levels helps you understand how different foods and lifestyle choices affect your body. Consult your healthcare provider for guidance on frequency and target ranges.
3. Carb Counting: Learning to count carbohydrates can empower you to make informed choices about your diet. Work with a registered dietitian to develop carb-counting skills and personalized meal plans.
4. Mindful Eating: Practicing mindful eating involves savoring each bite, eating slowly, and paying attention to hunger and fullness cues. This approach can prevent overeating and help manage blood sugar levels.
5. Physical Activity: Regular exercise improves insulin sensitivity and helps control blood sugar levels. Aim for a combination of aerobic exercise and strength training for optimal results.
6. Medication Management: If you're prescribed diabetes medications or insulin, work closely with your healthcare provider to ensure proper dosing and timing in relation to meals.
7. Weight Management: Losing excess weight, especially abdominal fat, can improve insulin sensitivity and blood sugar control. A registered dietitian can help you create a sustainable weight management plan.
8. Consistent Eating Schedule: Establishing regular eating times helps stabilize blood sugar levels and prevents extreme fluctuations.
9. Focus on Nutrient Density: Prioritize nutrient-dense foods that provide essential vitamins, minerals, and fiber. These foods support overall health and help manage blood sugar.
10. Individualized Approach: Diabetes management is highly individualized. Factors such as age, activity level, medication, and personal preferences influence dietary choices. Consulting a registered dietitian who specializes in diabetes can provide personalized guidance.

Preventing Type 2 Diabetes: Role of Nutrition

Type 2 diabetes is often preventable through lifestyle modifications, with nutrition playing a central role. Strategies for preventing type 2 diabetes include:

1. Healthy Eating Patterns: Adopting a diet rich in whole foods, vegetables, fruits, lean proteins, and whole grains can help maintain healthy blood sugar levels and prevent weight gain.
2. Moderate Carbohydrate Intake: Balancing carbohydrate intake with physical activity helps prevent blood sugar spikes. Choose complex carbohydrates and be mindful of portion sizes.
3. Weight Management: Maintaining a healthy weight through a balanced diet and regular physical activity significantly reduces the risk of developing type 2 diabetes.
4. Regular Exercise: Engaging in regular physical activity improves insulin sensitivity and supports weight management. Aim for at least 150 minutes of moderate-intensity exercise per week.

5. Limit Sugary Foods: Minimize sugary beverages, desserts, and processed foods to reduce the risk of insulin resistance and weight gain.
6. Hydration: Drinking water and non-caloric beverages instead of sugary drinks helps prevent excessive calorie intake and supports overall health.
7. Mindful Eating: Practicing mindful eating can prevent overeating and promote healthy food choices, contributing to diabetes prevention.
8. Regular Check-ups: Periodic medical check-ups can identify risk factors for diabetes, allowing for early intervention and prevention strategies.

Diabetes management and prevention hinge on the power of nutrition to regulate blood sugar levels, improve insulin sensitivity, and reduce complications. By understanding the role of carbohydrates, choosing nutrient-dense foods, practicing portion control, and adopting a balanced and mindful approach to eating, you can effectively manage diabetes and reduce the risk of complications. Remember that diabetes management and prevention are multifaceted endeavors that encompass nutrition, physical activity, medication management, and individualized care. Working closely with healthcare professionals, including registered dietitians and medical providers, empowers you to create a personalized plan that promotes your overall well-being and quality of life.

Chapter Five

Eating for Mental and Emotional Wellness

•*Brain-Boosting Foods for Cognitive Health*

Our brain, the epicenter of human intelligence and creativity, is a remarkable organ that constantly adapts, learns, and processes information. As we age, maintaining cognitive health becomes increasingly important, with concerns about memory, focus, and overall brain function. The foods we consume play a pivotal role in shaping our brain health, influencing cognitive performance and potentially reducing the risk of neurodegenerative diseases. This comprehensive guide explores the science behind brain-boosting foods, their impact on cognitive health, and effective strategies for nourishing the mind.

Understanding Cognitive Health: The Journey Across Lifespan

Understanding cognitive health across the lifespan is essential for promoting overall well-being and quality of life. Cognitive health refers to the ability to think, learn, remember, and make decisions. It encompasses various cognitive functions, including attention, memory, language, problem-solving, and executive functions.

Cognitive development begins in early childhood and continues throughout adulthood. In early childhood, the brain undergoes rapid growth and development, laying the foundation for cognitive skills. It is crucial to provide a nurturing and stimulating environment during this period to support optimal brain development. Activities that promote language development, problem-solving, and social interaction are particularly beneficial.

During adolescence, the brain undergoes significant changes, including synaptic pruning and myelination, which contribute to more efficient neural connections. However, the prefrontal cortex, responsible for executive functions such as decision-making and impulse control, continues to develop into early adulthood. Adolescents may benefit from activities that enhance cognitive skills, such as critical thinking, planning, and decision-making.

In adulthood, cognitive health is influenced by various factors, including lifestyle choices, genetics, and environmental factors. It is important to adopt healthy habits that support cognitive function. Regular physical exercise has been shown to have positive effects on cognitive health by increasing blood flow to the brain and promoting the growth of new neurons. A balanced diet that includes nutrient-rich foods, such as fruits, vegetables, whole grains, and healthy fats, also supports cognitive health.

Engaging in mentally stimulating activities, such as reading, puzzles, and learning new skills, can help maintain cognitive function and prevent cognitive decline. Social interaction and maintaining strong social connections are also important for cognitive health. Research has shown that social isolation and loneliness can negatively impact cognitive function.

As individuals age, they may experience changes in cognitive function. Mild cognitive impairment (MCI) is a condition characterized by noticeable memory or cognitive deficits that are greater than expected for age but do not interfere significantly with daily functioning. MCI can be a precursor to dementia, but not everyone with MCI will develop dementia. Early detection and intervention are crucial for managing MCI and potentially delaying the progression to dementia.

Promoting cognitive health in older adults involves a multifaceted approach. Regular physical exercise, a healthy diet, mental stimulation, social engagement, and managing chronic health conditions are all important factors. It is also important to address risk factors for cognitive decline, such as hypertension, diabetes, and smoking.

Overall, understanding cognitive health across the lifespan is essential for promoting optimal brain function and well-being. By adopting healthy lifestyle habits and engaging in activities that support cognitive function, individuals can enhance their cognitive health and potentially reduce the risk of cognitive decline and dementia.

The Role of Nutrition in Cognitive Health

Emerging research suggests that our dietary choices can profoundly impact cognitive health. Nutrients from foods interact with our brain's structure and function, influencing neural connections, neurotransmitter production, and inflammation levels. By incorporating brain-boosting foods into our diet, we can support cognitive function and potentially reduce the risk of cognitive decline and neurodegenerative diseases like Alzheimer's.

Nutrition plays a crucial role in cognitive health throughout the lifespan. A balanced diet that includes nutrient-rich foods provides the necessary fuel and building blocks for optimal brain function. Here are some key ways in which nutrition influences cognitive health:

1. Brain Development: During early childhood, proper nutrition is essential for optimal brain development. Nutrients like omega-3 fatty acids, iron, zinc, choline, and vitamins A, C, and E are particularly important. These nutrients support the growth and development of brain cells, neural connections, and myelin sheaths.
2. Memory and Learning: Certain nutrients have been found to enhance memory and learning abilities. For example, omega-3 fatty acids found in fatty fish, walnuts, and flaxseeds have been shown to improve cognitive function and reduce the risk of cognitive decline. Antioxidants found in fruits and vegetables, such as berries and leafy greens, protect brain cells from damage and improve memory.
3. Cognitive Decline: As individuals age, the risk of cognitive decline increases. However, a healthy diet can help slow down this process. Research suggests that a Mediterranean-style diet, rich in fruits, vegetables, whole grains, lean proteins, and healthy fats like olive oil and nuts, may lower the risk of cognitive decline and dementia.
4. Inflammation: Chronic inflammation has been linked to cognitive decline and neurodegenerative diseases like Alzheimer's disease. A diet high in processed foods,

   saturated fats, and added sugars can contribute to inflammation. On the other hand, a diet rich in anti-inflammatory foods like fruits, vegetables, whole grains, and healthy fats can help reduce inflammation and promote cognitive health.
5. Gut-Brain Connection: Emerging research has highlighted the importance of the gut-brain axis in cognitive health. The gut microbiome, which consists of trillions of bacteria in the digestive tract, plays a role in brain health and cognitive function. A healthy diet that includes fiber-rich foods, fermented foods, and probiotics can promote a diverse and balanced gut microbiome, which is beneficial for cognitive health.

It is important to note that nutrition is just one aspect of maintaining cognitive health. Other factors like physical exercise, mental stimulation, social interaction, and managing chronic health conditions also play a crucial role. A holistic approach that combines a healthy lifestyle with proper nutrition is key to promoting optimal cognitive function and reducing the risk of cognitive decline.

Key Nutrients for Cognitive Health

1. Omega-3 Fatty Acids: Found in fatty fish (salmon, mackerel, sardines), flaxseeds, chia seeds, and walnuts, omega-3 fatty acids are essential for brain health. They support neuronal structure, neurotransmitter function, and anti-inflammatory processes.
2. Antioxidants: These compounds, found in colorful fruits and vegetables, protect brain cells from oxidative stress and inflammation. Berries, leafy greens, and colorful peppers are rich sources of antioxidants.
3. B Vitamins: B vitamins, including B6, B12, and folate, play a role in neurotransmitter production and cognitive function. Leafy greens, legumes, eggs, and lean meats are good sources.
4. Vitamin D: Linked to brain health, vitamin D is found in fatty fish, fortified dairy products, and exposure to sunlight. Adequate levels are associated with better cognitive function.
5. Vitamin E: This antioxidant vitamin found in nuts, seeds, and vegetable oils helps protect cell membranes from damage.
6. Curcumin: The active compound in turmeric, curcumin has anti-inflammatory and antioxidant effects that may support cognitive health.
7. Iron: Iron is essential for oxygen transport and energy production in the brain. Lean meats, poultry, beans, and fortified cereals are iron-rich options.
8. Magnesium: Magnesium supports neuronal communication and may contribute to cognitive function. Spinach, nuts, seeds, and whole grains are magnesium sources.

Brain-Boosting Foods: Nourishing Cognitive Health

1. Fatty Fish: Fatty fish like salmon, mackerel, and sardines are rich in omega-3 fatty acids that support brain structure and function. Omega-3s may help reduce the risk of cognitive decline and improve mood.

2. Blueberries: Packed with antioxidants, blueberries have been dubbed "brain berries" for their potential to improve memory and cognitive function.
3. Leafy Greens: Spinach, kale, and Swiss chard provide a wealth of vitamins and minerals, including B vitamins, that support brain health.
4. Broccoli: Rich in antioxidants and vitamin K, broccoli may support cognitive health by reducing oxidative stress and inflammation.

5. Turmeric: Curcumin, the active compound in turmeric, has anti-inflammatory and antioxidant effects that may benefit brain health.
6. Pumpkin Seeds: High in magnesium, iron, zinc, and copper, pumpkin seeds contribute to overall brain function and health.
7. Dark Chocolate: Dark chocolate contains flavonoids that have been linked to improved cognitive function and enhanced blood flow to the brain.
8. Walnuts: Walnuts are a source of omega-3 fatty acids, antioxidants, and vitamin E, all of which contribute to brain health.
9. Eggs: Eggs are rich in choline, a nutrient that supports memory and cognitive function. They also provide high-quality protein.
10. Berries: Strawberries, raspberries, and blackberries contain antioxidants that protect brain cells and support cognitive function.

Strategies for Cognitive Health

1. Balanced Diet: Focus on a well-rounded diet that includes a variety of nutrient-dense foods to provide essential vitamins, minerals, and antioxidants.
2. Omega-3-Rich Foods: Regularly incorporate fatty fish, flaxseeds, chia seeds, and walnuts into your diet to ensure an adequate intake of omega-3 fatty acids.
3. Antioxidant-Rich Choices: Include colorful fruits and vegetables in every meal to provide a diverse array of antioxidants that protect brain cells.
4. Hydration: Staying hydrated supports overall brain function. Drink water and other hydrating beverages throughout the day.
5. Mindful Eating: Practice mindful eating to savor each bite, eat slowly, and recognize feelings of hunger and fullness.
6. Limit Processed Foods: Minimize processed foods high in added sugars and unhealthy fats, as they can contribute to inflammation and cognitive decline.
7. Healthy Fats: Choose healthy fats from sources like avocados, nuts, seeds, and olive oil to support brain health.
8. Limit Added Sugars: High sugar intake has been linked to cognitive decline. Minimize sugary snacks, desserts, and sugary beverages.
9. Whole Grains: Opt for whole grains like brown rice, quinoa, and whole wheat, which provide sustained energy and nutrients for brain health.
10. Regular Physical Activity: Engage in regular exercise, as it improves blood flow to the brain, enhances mood, and supports cognitive function.

11. Sleep Quality: Prioritize sufficient, restful sleep, as it's essential for memory consolidation and overall brain health.
12. Social Engagement: Maintaining social connections and engaging in stimulating activities can support cognitive health.

13. Mental Stimulation: Challenge your brain with activities like puzzles, games, reading, and learning new skills.
14. Stress Management: Chronic stress can negatively impact cognitive health. Practice stress-reduction techniques like meditation, deep breathing, and yoga.

The Mediterranean Diet: A Model for Cognitive Health

The Mediterranean diet is often highlighted as a model for brain-boosting nutrition due to its emphasis on whole foods, healthy fats,

Antioxidants, and omega-3-rich foods. This dietary pattern includes plenty of vegetables, fruits, whole grains, nuts, seeds, olive oil, and moderate consumption of fish and lean protein.

Research suggests that the Mediterranean diet is associated with improved cognitive function, reduced risk of cognitive decline, and a lower incidence of neurodegenerative diseases. Its focus on nutrient-dense, anti-inflammatory foods supports overall brain health.

Personalized Approach to Cognitive Health

Cognitive health is influenced by various factors, including genetics, lifestyle, medical history, and individual preferences. It's important to remember that no single food or diet can guarantee protection against cognitive decline. Instead, a combination of factors, including a balanced diet, regular physical activity, mental stimulation, stress management, and social engagement, contributes to cognitive well-being.

Consulting a healthcare professional or registered dietitian can provide personalized guidance based on your unique needs and goals. They can help you develop a dietary plan that aligns with your lifestyle and supports your journey toward optimal cognitive health.

A personalized approach to cognitive health takes into account an individual's unique nutritional needs, lifestyle factors, and health conditions. This approach recognizes that each person may have different dietary requirements and preferences, and therefore, tailors nutritional recommendations accordingly.

1. Nutritional Assessment: A personalized approach begins with a thorough assessment of an individual's current dietary habits, nutrient intake, and any specific nutritional deficiencies or imbalances. This assessment may involve analyzing dietary patterns, conducting blood tests to measure nutrient levels, and considering any existing health conditions or medications that may impact nutrient absorption or metabolism.

2. Individualized Nutrition Plan: Based on the assessment, a personalized nutrition plan is developed to address specific nutritional needs and goals. This plan may include

recommendations for specific foods, portion sizes, meal timings, and cooking methods to optimize nutrient intake. It may also involve supplementation if necessary to address any nutrient deficiencies.

3. Consideration of Health Conditions: Individuals with certain health conditions, such as diabetes, cardiovascular disease, or gastrointestinal disorders, may require specialized dietary approaches to support cognitive health. For example, a person with diabetes may need to focus on maintaining stable blood sugar levels to prevent cognitive impairment associated with high blood sugar fluctuations.

4. Lifestyle Factors: Personalized approaches also take into account lifestyle factors that can impact cognitive health. This may involve recommendations for regular physical exercise, stress management techniques, sleep hygiene practices, and strategies for managing mental health conditions like anxiety or depression. These lifestyle factors are important for overall brain health and can complement the effects of a balanced diet.

5. Regular Monitoring and Adjustments: A personalized approach to cognitive health recognizes that nutritional needs may change over time due to factors such as aging, hormonal changes, or shifts in health status. Regular monitoring of nutrient levels and cognitive function can help identify any necessary adjustments to the nutrition plan. This may involve periodic reassessment and modification of dietary recommendations.

In summary, a personalized approach to cognitive health acknowledges the individuality of nutritional needs and tailors recommendations accordingly. By considering factors such as current health status, dietary preferences, and lifestyle factors, this approach aims to optimize cognitive function and reduce the risk of cognitive decline on an individual level.

Brain-boosting foods offer a powerful strategy for promoting cognitive health and reducing the risk of cognitive decline. By incorporating nutrient-dense foods rich in omega-3 fatty acids, antioxidants, vitamins, and minerals, you can support brain structure and function. Combining a balanced diet with regular physical activity, mental stimulation, and stress management creates a holistic approach to nourishing your mind. Remember that cognitive health is a lifelong endeavor, and the choices you make today can have a positive impact on your cognitive function and well-being as you journey through life.

•*Mood-Enhancing Nutrients and Mental Resilience*

In the intricate tapestry of human emotions and mental well-being, the role of nutrition cannot be overlooked. Our dietary choices influence not only our physical health but also our mental state, mood, and emotional resilience. The connection between what we eat and how we feel is complex, with certain nutrients and dietary patterns showing the potential to enhance mood, support mental resilience, and even mitigate the risk of mood disorders. This comprehensive guide delves into the science behind mood-enhancing nutrients, their impact on mental health, and effective strategies for fostering emotional well-being.

Understanding the Mind-Body Connection

The intricate relationship between our mind and body has been recognized for centuries. Our mental state can influence our physical health, and vice versa. While external factors, life experiences, genetics, and brain chemistry contribute to our mental well-being, nutrition plays a significant role in shaping our mood and mental resilience.

The brain is a complex organ that requires a variety of nutrients to function optimally. Neurotransmitters, the chemical messengers that transmit signals in the brain, are influenced by the nutrients we consume. Imbalances in these neurotransmitters, such as serotonin, dopamine, and norepinephrine, are associated with mood disorders like depression and anxiety.

Mood-Enhancing Nutrients: Building Blocks of Emotional Well-Being

1. Omega-3 Fatty Acids: These essential fats, found in fatty fish (salmon, mackerel, sardines), flaxseeds, chia seeds, and walnuts, are integral to brain health. Omega-3s have anti-inflammatory properties and support the production of neurotransmitters involved in mood regulation.
2. B Vitamins: B vitamins, including B6, B12, and folate, are vital for neurotransmitter synthesis. They play a role in converting amino acids into mood-regulating neurotransmitters like serotonin and dopamine.
3. Magnesium: Magnesium is involved in hundreds of biochemical reactions, including those that impact mood regulation. Sources of magnesium include leafy greens, nuts, seeds, and whole grains.
4. Zinc: Zinc is essential for the production and regulation of neurotransmitters. It's found in foods like lean meats, poultry, legumes, and whole grains.
5. Vitamin D: Linked to mood disorders, vitamin D is synthesized in the skin in response to sunlight. Fatty fish, fortified dairy products, and supplementation are sources of this vital nutrient.
6. Antioxidants: Colorful fruits and vegetables are rich in antioxidants that protect brain cells from oxidative stress and inflammation, potentially influencing mood.

7. Amino Acids: Amino acids, the building blocks of proteins, play a role in neurotransmitter synthesis. Tryptophan, found in turkey, chicken, and nuts, is a precursor to serotonin.
8. Protein: Adequate protein intake supports the synthesis of neurotransmitters and helps stabilize blood sugar levels, which can impact mood.

Mood-Enhancing Foods: Nourishing Emotional Well-Being

1. Fatty Fish: Fatty fish like salmon, mackerel, and sardines provide omega-3 fatty acids that support brain health and mood regulation.
2. Leafy Greens: Spinach, kale, and Swiss chard offer a wealth of magnesium and other nutrients that contribute to mood balance.

3. Nuts and Seeds: Walnuts, flaxseeds, and chia seeds provide omega-3s, magnesium, and protein, all of which play a role in emotional well-being.
4. Berries: Berries are rich in antioxidants that protect brain cells from oxidative stress and inflammation, potentially influencing mood.
5. Whole Grains: Whole grains like brown rice, quinoa, and oats provide complex carbohydrates that support stable blood sugar levels and mood.
6. Lean Proteins: Lean meats, poultry, beans, and legumes offer amino acids that contribute to neurotransmitter synthesis and mood regulation.
7. Eggs: Eggs are a source of protein and contain tryptophan, a precursor to serotonin, a neurotransmitter linked to mood.
8. Dark Chocolate: Dark chocolate contains flavonoids that may enhance mood and improve blood flow to the brain.
9. Citrus Fruits: Citrus fruits like oranges and grapefruits provide vitamin C, which supports brain health and may influence mood.

Strategies for Fostering Emotional Well-Being

1. Balanced Diet: Prioritize a balanced diet that includes a variety of nutrient-dense foods to provide essential vitamins, minerals, and antioxidants.
2. Regular Meals: Maintain regular eating patterns to prevent blood sugar fluctuations, which can impact mood and energy levels.
3. Mindful Eating: Practice mindful eating by savoring each bite, eating slowly, and paying attention to hunger and fullness cues.
4. Hydration: Staying hydrated supports overall health and can impact mood and cognitive function.

5. Limit Processed Foods: Minimize processed foods high in added sugars, unhealthy fats, and artificial additives that can influence mood negatively.

6. Healthy Fats: Choose healthy fats from sources like avocados, nuts, seeds, and olive oil to support brain health and mood regulation.
7. Limit Added Sugars: High sugar intake can lead to energy crashes and mood swings. Minimize sugary snacks and desserts.
8. Physical Activity: Engaging in regular exercise promotes the release of endorphins, "feel-good" chemicals that enhance mood.
9. Sleep Quality: Prioritize sufficient, restful sleep, as sleep deprivation can impact mood and cognitive function.
10. Stress Management: Practice stress-reduction techniques like meditation, deep breathing, yoga, and spending time in nature.
11. Social Connection: Maintain meaningful social connections and engage in activities that bring joy and fulfillment.

12. Mental Stimulation: Challenge your brain with activities like puzzles, reading, learning new skills, and creative endeavors.
13. Seek Professional Support: If you're struggling with mood disorders like depression or anxiety, seek help from mental health professionals.

Creating a Mood-Boosting Lifestyle

Building mental resilience and fostering emotional well-being involves a holistic approach that extends beyond nutrition. While mood-enhancing nutrients and foods play a critical role, other lifestyle factors contribute to overall mental health:

1. Positive Mindset: Cultivate a positive outlook and practice gratitude to enhance mental resilience and emotional well-being.
2. Mindfulness and Meditation: Mindfulness practices and meditation help reduce stress, improve focus, and promote emotional balance.
3. Breathing Exercises: Deep breathing techniques can activate the relaxation response, reducing stress and promoting calmness.
4. Creative Outlets: Engage in creative activities that bring joy, such as painting, writing, playing a musical instrument, or crafting.
5. Social Support: Connect with loved ones, friends, and support groups to foster a sense of belonging and reduce feelings of isolation.
6. Nature and Physical Activity: Spending time in nature and engaging in physical activity can have profound positive effects on mood and mental resilience.
7. Professional Help: If you're struggling with persistent mood disturbances or mental health challenges, don't hesitate to seek help from mental health professionals.

Nurturing emotional well-being and building mental resilience are ongoing endeavors that encompass a multi-dimensional approach. While mood-enhancing nutrients and foods can positively influence brain chemistry and mood, lifestyle factors such as physical

Activity, stress management, social connection, and positive mindset are equally important. By incorporating mood-boosting foods, practicing mindful eating, embracing stress-reduction techniques, and seeking support when needed, you can foster emotional well-being and develop the mental resilience needed to navigate life's challenges with grace and positivity.

Chapter Six

Navigating Special Diets for Disease Management

•*Plant-Based and Vegetarian Diets: Benefits and Considerations*

The food choices we make have a profound impact on our health, the environment, and even ethical considerations. Plant-based and vegetarian diets are gaining popularity for their potential to improve health, reduce environmental footprint, and align with personal values. These dietary patterns emphasize plant-derived foods while limiting or excluding animal products. This comprehensive guide delves into the benefits and considerations of plant-based and vegetarian diets, offering insights into how these choices can impact health, the planet, and lifestyle.

Understanding Plant-Based and Vegetarian Diets

Plant-based and vegetarian diets share a common foundation of emphasizing plant-derived foods while varying in the degree of animal product exclusion:

1. Plant-Based Diet: A plant-based diet centers on plant-derived foods, such as fruits, vegetables, whole grains, legumes, nuts, and seeds. It minimizes or eliminates animal products but may include occasional consumption of animal-derived foods.
2. Vegetarian Diet: A vegetarian diet excludes meat, poultry, and seafood. However, it may include dairy products (lacto-vegetarian) or eggs (ovo-vegetarian). Some individuals choose lacto-ovo vegetarian diets, which include both dairy and eggs.
3. Vegan Diet: A vegan diet eliminates all animal products, including meat, dairy, eggs, and even honey. It is a strict plant-based diet that focuses solely on plant-derived foods.

Benefits of Plant-Based and Vegetarian Diets

- Health Benefits:
- Heart Health: Plant-based and vegetarian diets are associated with a reduced risk of heart disease. These diets are typically lower in saturated fats and cholesterol, promoting heart health.

- Weight Management: Plant-based diets tend to be lower in calorie density and higher in fiber, promoting weight loss and weight management.
- Blood Pressure: Plant-based diets, rich in potassium and antioxidants, can contribute to lower blood pressure levels.
- Diabetes Management: These diets may improve insulin sensitivity and blood sugar control, making them beneficial for individuals with type 2 diabetes.

- Reduced Risk of Chronic Diseases: Plant-based diets have been linked to a reduced risk of chronic diseases such as certain cancers, type 2 diabetes, and obesity.
- Environmental Benefits:
- Reduced Greenhouse Gas Emissions: Plant-based diets have a lower environmental footprint, as they require fewer resources and produce fewer greenhouse gas emissions compared to diets rich in animal products.
- Conservation of Resources: By consuming plant-based foods, fewer resources like water and land are required for food production, contributing to sustainability.
- Biodiversity Preservation: Plant-based diets promote biodiversity by reducing the demand for monoculture farming and animal agriculture.
- Ethical and Compassionate Considerations:
- Animal Welfare: Choosing plant-based and vegetarian diets aligns with ethical beliefs that prioritize animal welfare and reduce the demand for factory farming practices.
- Reduction of Animal Suffering: By excluding animal products, individuals contribute to the reduction of animal suffering associated with industrial farming.

Considerations and Potential Challenges

Nutritional Adequacy:
- Protein Intake: Plant-based diets can provide sufficient protein through sources like legumes, tofu, tempeh, nuts, seeds, and whole grains.
- Vitamin B12: Vitamin B12, primarily found in animal products, is crucial for nerve function and blood cell formation. Individuals on plant-based diets should consider supplementation or fortified foods.
- Omega-3 Fatty Acids: Plant-based sources of omega-3s include flaxseeds, chia seeds, walnuts, and algae-derived supplements.
- Iron and Calcium: While plant-based iron sources are available in leafy greens, beans, and fortified cereals, iron absorption can be improved by consuming vitamin C-rich foods. Calcium can be obtained from fortified plant-based milk, tofu, and leafy greens.

Meal Planning:

- Balanced Diet: To ensure nutritional adequacy, plan meals that include a variety of nutrient-dense plant-based foods from different food groups.

- Whole Foods: Prioritize whole, minimally processed foods over highly refined alternatives.

Potential Social and Practical Challenges:
- Social Situations: Dining out or attending social gatherings may require communication and planning to accommodate dietary preferences.

Family Considerations:
- If transitioning to a plant-based or vegetarian diet, family members' preferences and dietary needs should be considered.

Ethical and Cultural Factors:
- Personal Values: Plant-based and vegetarian diets may align with personal values related to animal welfare, environmental sustainability, and ethical beliefs.
- Cultural Traditions: Cultural and religious practices may influence dietary choices, and individuals can adapt plant-based diets to honor these traditions.

Creating a Balanced Plant-Based Diet

Variety and Diversity:
- Include a wide range of plant-derived foods, such as vegetables, fruits, whole grains, legumes, nuts, seeds, and plant-based proteins.

Protein-Rich Foods:
- Incorporate protein sources like beans, lentils, tofu, tempeh, seitan, quinoa, and nuts into your meals.

Whole Grains:
- Choose whole grains like brown rice, quinoa, oats, and whole wheat products for sustained energy and fiber.

Healthy Fats:
- Include sources of healthy fats like avocados, nuts, seeds, and olive oil to support brain health and overall well-being.

Fortified Foods:

- Include fortified plant-based milk, cereals, and nutritional yeast to ensure adequate intake of nutrients like calcium, vitamin B12, and iron.

Nutrient-Rich Snacks:

- Opt for nutrient-dense snacks like mixed nuts, hummus with veggies, fruit with nut butter, and whole-grain crackers.

Supplementation:

- Consider vitamin B12, vitamin D, and omega-3 supplements, especially if dietary intake is limited.

Making Informed Choices

- Gradual Transition: Consider gradually reducing animal products and increasing plant-based foods to allow your taste preferences and body to adjust.
- Listen to Your Body: Pay attention to hunger cues, energy levels, and how your body responds to different foods.
- Seek Professional Guidance: Consult a registered dietitian or healthcare provider for personalized guidance, especially if you have specific dietary needs or health conditions.

Plant-based and vegetarian diets offer a wealth of benefits for health, the environment, and ethical considerations. These dietary patterns can support heart health, weight management, chronic disease prevention, and contribute to a more sustainable planet. While considerations like nutritional adequacy, meal planning, and lifestyle adjustments may arise, they can be addressed through informed choices and strategic meal planning. Whether driven by health goals, environmental concerns, or ethical values, adopting a plant-based or vegetarian diet can be a powerful step toward promoting personal well-being and contributing to a more compassionate and sustainable world.

Gluten-Free, Dairy-Free, and Other Allergen-Free Approaches

For individuals with food allergies or sensitivities, the quest for a safe and nourishing diet is not just a matter of preference; it's a necessity. Gluten, dairy, and other common allergens can trigger a range of symptoms, from digestive distress to severe allergic reactions. In response, various allergen-free approaches have emerged, helping people manage their dietary needs while

enjoying a balanced and satisfying lifestyle. This comprehensive guide explores gluten-free, dairy-free, and other allergen-free diets, shedding light on their benefits, considerations, and strategies for creating wholesome and enjoyable meals.

Understanding Food Allergies and Sensitivities

Food allergies and sensitivities are immune responses triggered by specific proteins in certain foods. They can cause a range of symptoms, from mild discomfort to severe reactions. Common allergens include:

1. Gluten: A protein found in wheat, barley, and rye. People with celiac disease or non-celiac gluten sensitivity must avoid gluten to prevent adverse reactions.
2. Dairy: Dairy products contain lactose, a sugar that some people have difficulty digesting due to lactose intolerance. Others may be allergic to milk proteins.
3. Nuts: Tree nuts (such as almonds, walnuts, and cashews) and peanuts (a legume) are common allergens that can trigger severe reactions.
4. Soy: Soybeans and soy products can cause allergic reactions in some individuals.
5. Eggs: Egg allergies are common in children and may cause mild to severe symptoms.
6. Shellfish: Shellfish allergies can involve crustaceans (shrimp, crab, lobster) or mollusks (clams, mussels, oysters).
7. Fish: Fish allergies can range from mild to severe, and some people are allergic to certain types of fish.

Benefits of Allergen-Free Diets

1. Symptom Relief:
- Digestive Comfort: Avoiding trigger foods can alleviate digestive discomfort, bloating, and other gastrointestinal symptoms.
- Respiratory Relief: Allergen-free diets can improve respiratory symptoms in individuals with allergic reactions triggered by certain foods.
- Skin Health: For some individuals, eliminating allergens can lead to clearer skin and relief from conditions like eczema.

2. Disease Management:
- Celiac Disease: A gluten-free diet is essential for managing celiac disease, an autoimmune disorder that damages the small intestine in response to gluten consumption.
- Lactose Intolerance: Dairy-free diets are necessary for individuals with lactose intolerance, preventing digestive discomfort and symptoms.

3. Improved Well-Being:
- Enhanced Energy: Managing allergies can lead to increased energy levels and improved overall well-being.
- Mental Clarity: Relief from physical symptoms can contribute to mental clarity and focus.

Considerations and Potential Challenges

1. Nutritional Adequacy:
- Balanced Diet: Avoiding specific allergens requires careful planning to ensure a well-rounded, nutrient-dense diet.
- Nutrient Intake: Individuals with allergen restrictions may need to pay extra attention to nutrient intake, including protein, calcium, vitamin D, and B vitamins.

2. Meal Planning:
- Variety: Plan meals that incorporate a variety of allergen-free foods to ensure you're getting a wide range of nutrients.
- Whole Foods: Focus on whole, minimally processed foods to maximize nutritional value.

3. Social and Practical Challenges:
- Dining Out: Eating out can be challenging due to limited allergen-free options. Research menus and communicate your dietary needs with restaurant staff.
- Family Considerations: If your allergen-free diet differs from family members' diets, planning meals may require extra consideration.

4. Emotional Well-Being:
- Emotional Impact: Coping with dietary restrictions can sometimes be emotionally challenging. Seek support from friends, family, or support groups.

Creating a Balanced Allergen-Free Diet

1. Variety and Diversity: Include a wide range of allergen-free foods to ensure nutritional diversity.
2. Nutrient-Rich Foods: Incorporate nutrient-rich options like fruits, vegetables, whole grains, lean proteins, and healthy fats.
3. Protein Sources: Choose allergen-free protein sources such as legumes, beans, lentils, tofu, tempeh, seeds, and quinoa.
4. Calcium and Vitamin D: Include fortified plant-based milk alternatives or other fortified foods to ensure adequate calcium and vitamin D intake.

5. Healthy Fats: Incorporate sources of healthy fats like avocados, nuts, seeds, and olive oil.
6. Nutrient Supplements: Consult a healthcare provider or registered dietitian to determine if you need supplements to fill nutritional gaps.
7. Allergen-Free Baking: Experiment with allergen-free flours like almond flour, coconut flour, or gluten-free blends for baking.

Strategies for Successful Allergen-Free Living

1. Label Reading: Learn to read labels to identify potential allergens in packaged foods.
2. Recipe Adaptations: Adapt favorite recipes to be allergen-free by substituting ingredients or using allergen-free alternatives.
3. Meal Prep: Planning and prepping meals in advance can simplify allergen-free eating and save time.
4. Communication: When dining out or attending social gatherings, communicate your allergen restrictions with hosts or restaurant staff.
5. Support and Education: Seek support from online communities, forums, or local groups for individuals with similar dietary restrictions.
6. Professional Guidance: Consult a registered dietitian or healthcare provider to ensure your allergen-free diet meets your nutritional needs.

Allergen-free diets offer individuals with food allergies or sensitivities the opportunity to enjoy improved well-being and a higher quality of life. By identifying trigger foods and implementing allergen-free approaches, individuals can experience relief from uncomfortable symptoms and manage chronic conditions. While nutritional considerations, meal planning, and potential challenges may arise, a balanced and nutrient-rich diet can be achieved through careful planning, label reading, and the inclusion of a wide range of allergen-free foods. Whether motivated by health, symptom relief, or ethical values, adopting an allergen-free approach to eating can lead to a more fulfilling and enjoyable culinary journey.

Chapter Seven

The Gut-Health Connection

•*The Microbiome's Role in Disease Prevention and Immune Function*

Within the human body resides a vast ecosystem of microorganisms that collectively form the microbiome. This intricate community of bacteria, viruses, fungi, and other microbes plays a crucial role in maintaining health, influencing disease prevention, and regulating immune function. While once considered mere bystanders, these microbial inhabitants are now recognized as integral players in human well-being. This comprehensive exploration delves into the microbiome's significance in disease prevention, its impact on immune function, and the evolving understanding of its complex interactions within the body.

The Microbiome: An Ecosystem Within

The human body is host to trillions of microorganisms that reside in various niches, including the skin, oral cavity, and most notably, the gastrointestinal tract. Collectively, these microorganisms form a dynamic and complex ecosystem known as the microbiome. This intricate community collaborates with the human host in ways that influence metabolism, digestion, immune responses, and overall health.

The microbiome refers to the collection of microorganisms, including bacteria, viruses, fungi, and other microbes, that live in and on our bodies. It is often referred to as an ecosystem within our bodies because it plays a crucial role in maintaining our overall health and well-being.

1. Composition of the Microbiome: The microbiome is highly diverse, with trillions of microorganisms residing in different parts of our bodies, such as the gut, skin, mouth, and reproductive organs. Each person's microbiome is unique, influenced by factors such as genetics, diet, lifestyle, and environmental exposures.

2. Gut-Brain Connection: The gut microbiome, in particular, has been linked to cognitive health through the gut-brain axis. The gut and the brain communicate bidirectionally through various pathways, including neural, hormonal, and immune signaling. The composition and activity of the gut microbiome can influence brain function and behavior, including cognition, mood, and stress responses.

3. Impact on Neurotransmitters: The microbiome produces various neurotransmitters and metabolites that can influence brain function. For example, certain bacteria in the gut produce

neurotransmitters like serotonin and dopamine, which play key roles in regulating mood and cognitive function. Imbalances in these neurotransmitters due to disruptions in the microbiome have been associated with conditions such as depression and anxiety.

4. Immune System Regulation: The microbiome also plays a critical role in regulating the immune system. It helps educate and train the immune system to recognize and respond appropriately to pathogens while maintaining tolerance to harmless substances. Imbalances in the gut microbiome have been linked to immune dysregulation and inflammatory conditions, which can impact cognitive health.

5. Influence on Nutrient Metabolism: The microbiome is involved in the digestion and metabolism of nutrients from our diet. It helps break down complex carbohydrates, fibers, and other components that our own digestive enzymes cannot fully process. This process produces short-chain fatty acids, which are important energy sources for the cells lining the gut and have been shown to support brain health.

6. Role in Neurodegenerative Diseases: Emerging research suggests that alterations in the microbiome may contribute to the development and progression of neurodegenerative diseases such as Alzheimer's disease and Parkinson's disease. Imbalances in the gut microbiome have been associated with increased inflammation, oxidative stress, and the accumulation of abnormal proteins in the brain, all of which are implicated in these diseases.

7. Modulation of the Microbiome: The composition and diversity of the microbiome can be influenced by various factors, including diet, medications (such as antibiotics), stress, and environmental exposures. Certain dietary components, such as fiber-rich foods, prebiotics, and probiotics, can promote a healthy and diverse microbiome. Lifestyle factors, such as regular exercise and stress management, can also positively impact the microbiome.

In conclusion, the microbiome is an intricate ecosystem within our bodies that plays a vital role in cognitive health. Understanding the interactions between the microbiome and the brain can lead to personalized approaches that optimize the microbiome's composition and function, promoting cognitive well-being and potentially reducing the risk of neurodegenerative diseases.

The Gut Microbiome: A Hub of Activity

The gut microbiome refers to the collection of microorganisms, including bacteria, viruses, fungi, and other microbes, that reside in the gastrointestinal tract. It is often described as a "hub of activity" due to its crucial role in various physiological processes and its impact on overall health.

The gut microbiome is incredibly diverse, with trillions of microorganisms present. These microbes play a vital role in digestion, nutrient absorption, and metabolism. They break down complex carbohydrates, fibers, and other indigestible substances that our own digestive enzymes

cannot process. In return, they produce short-chain fatty acids and vitamins that are beneficial to our health.

Beyond digestion, the gut microbiome also plays a critical role in regulating the immune system. The presence of beneficial bacteria helps train and modulate the immune response, preventing inappropriate immune reactions and reducing the risk of autoimmune diseases. Additionally, the gut microbiome acts as a barrier against harmful pathogens by competing for resources and producing antimicrobial substances.

Moreover, emerging research suggests that the gut microbiome has a significant impact on mental health and brain function. The gut-brain axis, a bidirectional communication system between the gut and the brain, allows the microbiome to influence mood, behavior, and cognitive function. Imbalances in the gut microbiome have been associated with conditions such as anxiety, depression, and neurodegenerative diseases.

Furthermore, the gut microbiome has been linked to metabolic disorders such as obesity and type 2 diabetes. Certain microbial compositions have been found to be associated with increased energy extraction from food and increased fat storage. Conversely, a diverse and healthy gut microbiome is associated with better weight management and metabolic health.

Factors such as diet, lifestyle, medications (especially antibiotics), stress, and environmental exposures can influence the composition and diversity of the gut microbiome. A diet rich in fiber and plant-based foods promotes microbial diversity, while a diet high in processed foods and low in fiber can lead to a less diverse and less healthy microbiome.

In recent years, there has been growing interest in manipulating the gut microbiome to improve health outcomes. Probiotics, which are live microorganisms that confer health benefits when consumed, have gained popularity as a means to improve gut health. Additionally, fecal microbiota transplantation (FMT) has shown promising results in treating certain gut-related disorders, such as Clostridium difficile infection.

In conclusion, the gut microbiome is a dynamic and complex ecosystem that plays a crucial role in various aspects of human health. Its influence extends beyond digestion and metabolism to immune function, mental health, and metabolic disorders. Understanding and harnessing the potential of the gut microbiome may lead to new therapeutic approaches and interventions for a wide range of health conditions.

Disease Prevention and the Microbiome

1. Immune System Education:

   - Early Exposure: During infancy and early childhood, exposure to various microbes helps educate the developing immune system. This exposure aids in distinguishing between harmless and harmful agents, reducing the risk of inappropriate immune responses.

   - Tolerance Development: The presence of a diverse and balanced microbiome helps promote immune tolerance, preventing unnecessary immune reactions against innocuous substances.

2. Protection Against Pathogens:

   - Competitive Exclusion: A healthy microbiome can outcompete pathogenic microorganisms for resources, limiting their ability to establish themselves and cause infections.

   - Production of Antimicrobial Substances: Some microorganisms within the microbiome produce antimicrobial substances that inhibit the growth of harmful pathogens.

3. Inflammatory and Autoimmune Disease Prevention:

   - Gut Barrier Integrity: A balanced microbiome contributes to the maintenance of the gut barrier, preventing the translocation of harmful substances and potential triggers for inflammation.

   - Anti-Inflammatory Effects: Certain microbial metabolites can have anti-inflammatory effects, potentially reducing the risk of chronic inflammatory diseases.

Immune Function and the Microbiome

1. Immune System Maturation:

   - Immunoglobulin A (IgA) Production: The gut microbiome influences the production of IgA antibodies, which play a critical role in immune defense at mucosal surfaces.

   - Immune Cell Development: Microbial exposure in early life helps shape the development and function of immune cells, ensuring a balanced immune response.

2. Immune Activation and Regulation:

   - Tolerogenic Responses: The gut microbiome helps induce tolerogenic responses that prevent excessive immune activation against harmless antigens.

   - Regulatory T Cells: Some gut bacteria promote the differentiation of regulatory T cells, which help modulate immune responses and prevent autoimmune reactions.

3. Disease Susceptibility and Immune Modulation:

   - Links to Chronic Diseases: Imbalances in the gut microbiome have been associated with various chronic diseases, including autoimmune disorders, allergies, and metabolic conditions.

   - Microbial Metabolites: Microbes produce metabolites that can directly influence immune cell behavior, impacting disease susceptibility.

4. Impact of Antibiotics:

   - Antibiotics and Microbiome Disruption: Broad-spectrum antibiotics can disrupt the balance of the gut microbiome, potentially leading to immune dysregulation and increased susceptibility to infections.

Personalized Microbiome Health

1. Dietary Influences:

   - Prebiotic Fiber: Consuming foods rich in prebiotic fibers (found in fruits, vegetables, and whole grains) can support the growth of beneficial gut bacteria.

   - Fermented Foods: Fermented foods like yogurt, kefir, sauerkraut, and kimchi contain live beneficial bacteria that can contribute to a healthy gut microbiome.

2. Antibiotics and Medications:

- Responsible Antibiotic Use: When antibiotics are necessary, healthcare providers aim to prescribe them judiciously to minimize disruption of the microbiome.

- Probiotics: Some individuals may benefit from probiotic supplements to restore gut microbial balance after antibiotic treatment.

3. Lifestyle Factors:

- Stress Management: Chronic stress can impact the gut-brain axis and influence the composition of the gut microbiome. Stress management techniques may help maintain a balanced microbiome.

- Physical Activity: Regular exercise has been associated with a more diverse gut microbiome and improved immune function.

4. Microbiome Testing:

- Microbiome analysis services are available to provide insights into the composition of an individual's microbiome. However, interpretation of results is complex and evolving.

Future Frontiers in Microbiome Research

1. Precision Medicine: As research advances, personalized approaches to microbiome health may become more common, tailoring recommendations based on an individual's unique microbial composition.

2. Therapeutic Potential: Microbiome-targeted therapies, including probiotics, prebiotics, and microbial transplants, are being explored for their potential to treat various diseases and conditions.

3. Unraveling Microbial Interactions: Ongoing research aims to understand the intricate interactions between different microbial species and how they collectively influence health and disease.

The microbiome's role in disease prevention and immune function is a rapidly evolving area of research that continues to unveil the remarkable influence of microbial inhabitants within the human body. From shaping immune responses to promoting tolerance and preventing infections, the microbiome's impact is extensive and multifaceted. As scientific understanding deepens, harnessing the potential of the microbiome to enhance disease prevention and support immune function offers a promising avenue for improving human health and well-being.

•Probiotics, Prebiotics, and Gut-Healing Foods

Within the intricate landscape of the human body, a diverse community of microorganisms resides, collectively known as the microbiome. This bustling ecosystem, particularly prominent in the gut, plays a vital role in maintaining health, supporting digestion, and regulating immune responses. Probiotics, prebiotics, and specific gut-healing foods have emerged as key players in promoting the health and balance of this microbial community. This exploration delves into the significance of probiotics, the importance of prebiotics, and the nurturing power of gut-healing foods in maintaining a well-functioning microbiome.

Understanding Probiotics: Nature's Health Allies

Probiotics are live microorganisms that, when consumed in adequate amounts, confer health benefits to the host. Often referred to as "good bacteria," probiotics can help restore and maintain a balanced gut microbiome, promoting optimal digestion and immune function.

Types of Probiotics:

- Lactic Acid Bacteria: Lactobacillus and Bifidobacterium are common strains of lactic acid bacteria found in many probiotic supplements and fermented foods.
- Yeasts: Saccharomyces boulardii is a yeast strain often used as a probiotic to support gut health.

Health Benefits of Probiotics:

- Digestive Health: Probiotics aid in breaking down food, enhancing nutrient absorption, and preventing digestive discomfort.
- Immune Function: A well-balanced gut microbiome influenced by probiotics supports a robust immune response.
- Gut Barrier Integrity: Probiotics help maintain the integrity of the gut lining, preventing the translocation of harmful substances.
- Inflammatory Responses: Some probiotics produce anti-inflammatory compounds that may reduce the risk of chronic inflammatory diseases.

Prebiotics: Fueling Microbial Harmony

Prebiotics are non-digestible fibers found in certain foods that serve as nourishment for beneficial gut bacteria. By providing sustenance to these microbes, prebiotics help them flourish and contribute to a balanced microbiome.

Types of Prebiotics:

- Inulin: Found in foods like chicory root, garlic, onions, and asparagus, inulin promotes the growth of beneficial bacteria.
- Fructooligosaccharides (FOS): Similar to inulin, FOS is abundant in foods like bananas, leeks, and artichokes.
- Resistant Starch: Found in legumes, green bananas, and cooked and cooled potatoes, resistant starch supports gut health.

Benefits of Prebiotics:

- Microbial Diversity: Prebiotics help maintain a diverse range of gut bacteria, supporting a thriving microbiome.

- Bifidobacteria Growth: Certain prebiotics selectively promote the growth of beneficial Bifidobacteria.
- Short-Chain Fatty Acids: As beneficial bacteria consume prebiotics, they produce short-chain fatty acids that benefit gut health.

Gut-Healing Foods: Nourishing from Within

Gut-healing foods are those that promote a healthy gut microbiome and support the overall health of the gastrointestinal tract. These foods are often rich in fiber, antioxidants, and beneficial nutrients that nourish the gut and provide a favorable environment for the growth of beneficial bacteria.

One example of a gut-healing food is fermented foods. Fermented foods such as yogurt, kefir, sauerkraut, and kimchi contain live bacteria that can help populate the gut with beneficial microbes. These probiotic-rich foods can improve digestion, enhance nutrient absorption, and support a healthy immune system.

Another category of gut-healing foods is prebiotics. Prebiotics are non-digestible fibers that serve as food for the beneficial bacteria in the gut. They can be found in foods such as onions, garlic, leeks, asparagus, bananas, and whole grains. Consuming prebiotic-rich foods can help stimulate the growth of beneficial bacteria and promote a healthy balance in the gut microbiome.

In addition to fermented foods and prebiotics, other gut-healing foods include bone broth, which is rich in collagen and amino acids that support gut health and repair the intestinal lining. Ginger and turmeric are also known for their anti-inflammatory properties, which can help reduce inflammation in the gut and promote healing.

Furthermore, incorporating a variety of fruits and vegetables into the diet is essential for gut health. These plant-based foods are high in fiber, antioxidants, and phytochemicals, all of which support a healthy gut microbiome and provide essential nutrients for optimal digestion and overall health.

It's important to note that individual responses to different foods may vary, and what works for one person may not work for another. It's always best to listen to your body and pay attention to how certain foods make you feel. Consulting with a healthcare professional or registered dietitian can also provide personalized guidance on gut-healing foods based on individual needs and health conditions.

Gut-healing foods are those that promote a healthy gut microbiome and support overall gut health. Incorporating fermented foods, prebiotics, bone broth, ginger, turmeric, and a variety of fruits and vegetables into the diet can help nourish the gut from within and support optimal digestive function and overall well-being.

Creating a Gut-Healing Approach

- Incorporate Variety: Consume a diverse range of foods to support a diverse microbiome.
- Whole Foods Focus: Choose whole, minimally processed foods to maximize nutrient intake and nourish the microbiome.
- Prebiotic-Rich Choices: Include prebiotic foods like onions, garlic, asparagus, and bananas in your meals.
- Probiotic Inclusions: Integrate fermented foods like yogurt, kefir, sauerkraut, and kimchi into your diet.

- Mindful Eating: Practice mindful eating to aid digestion and enhance nutrient absorption.
- Hydration: Stay hydrated to support overall digestion and gut function.
- Limit Processed Foods: Minimize processed foods high in added sugars and unhealthy fats, as they can negatively impact gut health.
- Lifestyle Considerations: Manage stress, engage in regular physical activity, and prioritize sufficient sleep for overall well-being.

Probiotics, prebiotics, and gut-healing foods collectively contribute to a thriving and balanced microbiome, which in turn supports digestive health, immune function, and overall well-being. By incorporating these components into your dietary approach, you can create an environment within your body that fosters the growth of beneficial bacteria, enhances nutrient absorption, and reduces inflammation. As research continues to uncover the intricate connections between the gut microbiome and various aspects of health, embracing a diet rich in probiotics, prebiotics, and gut-healing foods becomes a proactive step toward nurturing your body's internal ecosystem and promoting optimal vitality.

Chapter Eight

Overcoming Challenges and Making Lasting Changes

•*Strategies for Overcoming Food Cravings and Unhealthy Habits*

Food cravings and unhealthy habits are common challenges that many individuals face on their journey toward a healthier lifestyle. The allure of sugary snacks, fast food, and comfort foods can often overpower our best intentions, leading to unhealthy eating patterns. However, with the right strategies and a proactive mindset, it is possible to overcome these cravings and habits and establish a more balanced approach to eating. This comprehensive guide explores the underlying factors of food cravings, the psychology of unhealthy habits, and actionable strategies for making positive changes that support long-term well-being.

Understanding Food Cravings: The Science Behind the Desire

To effectively overcome food cravings and unhealthy habits, it is important to understand the underlying causes. Cravings can be triggered by various factors, including emotional states, physiological imbalances, social cues, and learned behaviors. Emotional cravings are often linked to stress, boredom, sadness, or other emotional states. Physiological imbalances can be caused by nutrient deficiencies or hormonal fluctuations. Social cues, such as seeing others eat certain foods or being in specific environments, can also trigger cravings. Lastly, learned behaviors refer to the association between certain foods and pleasurable experiences. By identifying the root causes of cravings, individuals can better address them and find alternative ways to satisfy their needs.

1. Biological Factors:

   - Brain Reward System: Certain foods, particularly those high in sugar and fat, activate the brain's reward system, triggering the release of dopamine and creating a sense of pleasure and satisfaction.

   - Hormonal Influence: Hormones like ghrelin (the hunger hormone) and leptin (the satiety hormone) can influence appetite and food cravings.

2. Psychological Factors:

   - Emotional Eating: Emotions, stress, boredom, and other psychological triggers can lead to food cravings as a way to cope with feelings.

   - Food Associations: Positive memories and associations with certain foods can trigger cravings for comfort and nostalgia.

3. Environmental Factors:

   - Food Advertising: Exposure to advertisements and images of unhealthy foods can stimulate cravings.

   - Availability: The accessibility of high-calorie, highly palatable foods can increase the likelihood of cravings.

Breaking Unhealthy Habits: The Power of Mindset

Unhealthy habits are behaviors that undermine well-being and health goals. They can be deeply ingrained and challenging to change. Understanding the psychological mechanisms behind habits and adopting a proactive mindset are key to overcoming them.

1. Habit Loop:

   - Cue: Triggers that prompt the habit, such as stress, time of day, or location.

   - Routine: The behavior itself, which could be unhealthy eating or another detrimental action.

   - Reward: The positive feeling or outcome associated with the behavior, which reinforces its repetition.

2. Mindfulness and Self-Awareness:

   - Recognize Triggers: Identifying the cues that lead to unhealthy habits can help you proactively address them.

   - Self-Reflect: Understand the emotional and psychological factors that contribute to habit formation.

3. Cognitive Behavioral Strategies:

   - Cognitive Restructuring: Challenge and reframe negative thought patterns that contribute to unhealthy habits.

   - Substitution: Replace an unhealthy habit with a healthier alternative to satisfy the same need or desire.

   - Positive Reinforcement: Reward yourself for making positive changes, reinforcing new habits.

Actionable Strategies for Overcoming Cravings and Habits

1. Develop a Balanced Eating Plan:

Create a meal plan that includes nutrient-dense foods to satisfy hunger and prevent extreme cravings.

Include Protein and Fiber: Protein-rich foods and high-fiber sources help keep you full and stabilize blood sugar levels.

2. Mindful Eating:

Mindful eating is a powerful strategy for overcoming food cravings and unhealthy habits. It involves paying full attention to the present moment while eating, including the taste, smell, texture, and sensations of each bite. By practicing mindfulness, individuals can become more aware of their body's hunger and fullness cues, making it easier to distinguish between true hunger and emotional cravings. Mindful eating also helps individuals savor their food and derive more satisfaction from smaller portions. Techniques such as eating slowly, chewing thoroughly, and putting down utensils between bites can enhance the mindful eating experience.

3. Hydration:

Drink Water: Staying hydrated can reduce the intensity of cravings and help prevent mistaking thirst for hunger.

4. Manage Stress:

Stress is a common trigger for food cravings and unhealthy habits. When stressed, individuals often turn to food as a way to cope or find comfort. Therefore, managing stress is an essential strategy for overcoming cravings. Engaging in stress-reducing activities such as exercise, meditation, deep breathing, or hobbies can help individuals find healthier ways to manage stress and reduce the likelihood of turning to food for comfort. Additionally, seeking support from friends, family, or professionals can provide individuals with the tools and techniques needed to effectively manage stress.

5. Sleep Well:

Prioritize Sleep: Aim for 7-9 hours of quality sleep per night to regulate hormones that influence hunger and cravings.

6. Balanced Snacking:

Choose Nutrient-Dense Snacks: Opt for fruits, vegetables, nuts, and yogurt to satisfy between-meal hunger.

7. Plan Indulgences:

Allow Treats: Incorporate occasional treats into your eating plan to avoid feelings of deprivation.

Practice Moderation: Enjoy indulgent foods mindfully and in reasonable portions.

8. Create a Supportive Environment:

Creating a supportive environment is crucial for overcoming food cravings and unhealthy habits. This includes surrounding oneself with people who support healthy choices and avoiding environments that trigger cravings. For example, individuals can seek out friends or family members who have similar health goals and engage in activities that do not revolve around food. Additionally, removing unhealthy foods from the home and stocking it with nutritious options can help reduce temptation. Creating a supportive environment also involves planning meals and snacks in advance, so individuals are less likely to rely on unhealthy options when hunger strikes.

9. Stay Active:

Regular Exercise: Engage in physical activity, as it can help regulate appetite and improve mood.

10. Seek Professional Help:

In some cases, overcoming food cravings and unhealthy habits may require professional help. Registered dietitians, therapists, or counselors can provide guidance and support tailored to individual needs. These professionals can help individuals identify the root causes of cravings, develop personalized strategies, and address any underlying emotional or psychological factors that contribute to unhealthy habits. Seeking professional help is especially important for individuals with eating disorders or those who struggle with severe cravings that significantly impact their daily life and well-being.

11. Set Realistic Goals:

Focus on Progress: Celebrate small victories and gradual changes as you work toward healthier habits.

12. Practice Self-Compassion:

Be Kind to Yourself: Avoid self-criticism if you slip up and focus on getting back on track.

Overcoming food cravings and unhealthy habits requires a combination of knowledge, self-awareness, and actionable strategies. By understanding the underlying factors of cravings and habits, adopting a proactive mindset, and implementing practical techniques, you can take charge of your eating habits and make positive changes that support your well-being. Remember that progress is a journey, and each step you take toward balanced eating and healthier habits brings you closer to a more vibrant and fulfilling lifestyle.

•*Sustaining Positive Dietary Changes for Long-Term Health*

Sustaining positive dietary changes for long-term health is a crucial aspect of maintaining a healthy lifestyle. Many individuals struggle with making dietary changes due to various reasons, such as lack of motivation, difficulty in breaking old habits, or the temptation to revert to unhealthy eating patterns. However, with the right strategies and mindset, it is possible to sustain positive dietary changes and reap the long-term health benefits. In this article, we will discuss various strategies for sustaining positive dietary changes for long-term health, including setting realistic goals, making gradual changes, finding enjoyment in healthy foods, developing a meal planning routine, seeking support, practicing self-compassion, and staying motivated.

Setting Realistic Goals:

Setting realistic goals is essential for sustaining positive dietary changes for long-term health. It is important to set goals that are achievable and align with individual capabilities and preferences. Unrealistic goals can lead to frustration and disappointment, making it more likely for individuals to give up on their dietary changes. For example, instead of aiming to completely eliminate all unhealthy foods from one's diet, a more realistic goal could be to reduce the consumption of unhealthy foods and increase the intake of nutritious options. By setting small, attainable goals, individuals can gradually make sustainable changes that are easier to maintain in the long run.

Making Gradual Changes:

Making gradual changes is another effective strategy for sustaining positive dietary changes for long-term health. Instead of completely overhauling one's diet overnight, it is often more sustainable to make small, incremental changes over time. This allows individuals to adjust to the new dietary habits and develop a sense of familiarity and comfort with healthier options. For example, instead of eliminating all sugary beverages at once, individuals can start by replacing one sugary drink with water or a healthier alternative each day. Gradual changes also help prevent feelings of deprivation or restriction, making it easier to stick with the new dietary habits.

Finding Enjoyment in Healthy Foods:

Finding enjoyment in healthy foods is crucial for sustaining positive dietary changes for long-term health. Many individuals associate healthy eating with bland, tasteless meals, which can make it challenging to stick with a nutritious diet. However, healthy eating can be both delicious and satisfying with the right approach. Experimenting with different cooking techniques, flavors,

and spices can help individuals discover new ways to make healthy foods more enjoyable. Additionally, incorporating favorite fruits, vegetables, or whole grains into meals can add familiarity and increase the likelihood of sustaining positive dietary changes.

Developing a Meal Planning Routine:

Developing a meal planning routine is a practical strategy for sustaining positive dietary changes for long-term health. Meal planning involves organizing and preparing meals and snacks in advance, which helps individuals make healthier choices and avoid impulsive or unhealthy food choices. By planning meals ahead of time, individuals can ensure that they have nutritious options readily available and reduce the reliance on convenience or fast foods. Meal planning also allows individuals to incorporate a variety of foods from different food groups, ensuring a balanced and nutrient-rich diet.

Seeking Support:

Seeking support is an important strategy for sustaining positive dietary changes for long-term health. It can be challenging to make dietary changes alone, especially when faced with social pressures or temptations. Therefore, seeking support from friends, family members, or support groups can provide individuals with the encouragement and accountability needed to stay on track. Sharing goals and progress with others can also create a sense of community and motivation. Additionally, seeking professional help from registered dietitians or nutritionists can provide i ndividuals with personalized guidance and support tailored to their specific needs.

Practicing Self-Compassion:

Practicing self-compassion is a crucial strategy for sustaining positive dietary changes for long-term health. It is common for individuals to experience setbacks or slip-ups along their journey towards healthier eating habits. Instead of being overly critical or judgmental towards oneself, it is important to practice self-compassion and view setbacks as learning opportunities. Being kind and forgiving towards oneself can help individuals bounce back from setbacks and continue making positive dietary changes. It is essential to remember that sustaining positive dietary changes is a long-term process, and it is normal to face challenges along the way.

Staying Motivated:

Staying motivated is a key strategy for sustaining positive dietary changes for long-term health. Motivation can fluctuate over time, making it important to find strategies that help maintain enthusiasm and commitment towards healthy eating habits. One effective strategy is to set short-term rewards or incentives for achieving dietary goals. For example, treating oneself to a non-food reward, such as a spa day or a new workout outfit, can provide motivation and reinforce

positive behaviors. Additionally, tracking progress and celebrating small victories can help individuals stay motivated and focused on their long-term health goals.

Sustaining positive dietary changes for long-term health requires dedication, perseverance, and a willingness to make lasting changes. By setting realistic goals, making gradual changes, finding enjoyment in healthy foods, developing a meal planning routine, seeking support, practicing self-compassion, and staying motivated, individuals can sustain positive dietary changes and improve their long-term health outcomes. It is important to remember that everyone's journey is unique, and what works for one person may not work for another. Therefore, it is essential to listen to one's body, experiment with different strategies, and find a personalized approach that works best for long-term success in maintaining a healthy lifestyle.

Chapter Nine

Nutrient-Packed Meals and Snacks for Disease Prevention

•*Nutrient-Packed Meals and Snacks for Disease Prevention*

In the pursuit of optimal health and disease prevention, the role of nutrition cannot be overstated. A diet rich in nutrient-packed meals and snacks plays a crucial role in supporting the body's defenses, enhancing immune function, and reducing the risk of chronic diseases. By making intentional choices to include a diverse range of vitamins, minerals, antioxidants, and other essential nutrients, individuals can empower themselves to lead a healthier and more fulfilling life. This comprehensive exploration delves into the importance of nutrient-packed foods, strategies for creating balanced meals and snacks, and their significant impact on disease prevention and overall well-being.

Understanding Nutrient-Packed Foods

Nutrient-packed foods, often referred to as nutrient-dense foods, are those that provide a high concentration of essential nutrients relative to their calorie content. These foods are rich in vitamins, minerals, antioxidants, fiber, and other bioactive compounds that play a vital role in maintaining bodily functions, supporting metabolism, and protecting against diseases.

1. Vitamins and Minerals: Vitamins such as A, C, D, and E, along with minerals like calcium, magnesium, and iron, are critical for various physiological processes.

2. Antioxidants: Antioxidants, found in colorful fruits and vegetables, help neutralize harmful free radicals and reduce oxidative stress, which is associated with chronic diseases.

3. Fiber: Dietary fiber, present in whole grains, legumes, fruits, and vegetables, supports digestive health, regulates blood sugar levels, and promotes a feeling of fullness.

4. Healthy Fats: Essential fatty acids like omega-3s and omega-6s are crucial for brain health, inflammation regulation, and cardiovascular function.

5. Phytonutrients: Phytonutrients, found in plant-based foods, have various health benefits and contribute to the prevention of chronic diseases.

Strategies for Creating Nutrient-Packed Meals

1. Balanced Macronutrients: Incorporate a variety of nutrient-dense foods from all macronutrient categories: carbohydrates, proteins, and fats.

2. Colorful Produce: Fill your plate with a rainbow of fruits and vegetables to ensure a diverse intake of vitamins, minerals, and antioxidants.

3. Lean Proteins: Opt for lean protein sources such as poultry, fish, legumes, tofu, and nuts to support muscle health and metabolism.

4. Whole Grains: Choose whole grains like quinoa, brown rice, whole wheat, and oats for sustained energy and fiber.

5. Healthy Fats: Include sources of healthy fats such as avocados, nuts, seeds, and olive oil to support heart health and nutrient absorption.

6. Mindful Portion Control: Pay attention to portion sizes to avoid overeating while still getting essential nutrients.

7. Hydration: Drink plenty of water throughout the day to support digestion and overall bodily functions.

8. Homemade Meals: Prepare meals at home to have control over ingredients and cooking methods, reducing unnecessary additives and excess sodium.

Nutrient-Packed Snacking Strategies

1. Protein-Rich Snacks: Choose snacks that contain protein, such as Greek yogurt, cottage cheese, or nut butter, to keep you full and satisfied.

2. Fruit and Vegetable Snacks: Enjoy fruits and vegetables with hummus, yogurt dip, or a small amount of nut butter for added nutrients.

3. Nuts and Seeds: Nuts and seeds are rich in healthy fats, fiber, and essential nutrients, making them a satisfying and nutrient-packed snack.

4. Whole Grain Snacks: Opt for whole grain crackers, rice cakes, or popcorn for a fiber-rich and energizing snack.

5. Hydration: Include herbal teas, infused water, or water-rich fruits like watermelon for hydration between meals.

Impact on Disease Prevention

1. Cardiovascular Health: Nutrient-packed foods rich in antioxidants, fiber, and healthy fats support heart health by reducing inflammation, regulating blood pressure, and improving cholesterol levels.

2. Type 2 Diabetes Prevention: A diet high in fiber, whole grains, and nutrient-dense foods can help regulate blood sugar levels and reduce the risk of type 2 diabetes.

3. Cancer Prevention: Antioxidant-rich foods, such as berries, cruciferous vegetables, and leafy greens, help protect cells from DNA damage and lower the risk of certain cancers.

4. Bone Health: Nutrient-packed foods rich in calcium, vitamin D, magnesium, and vitamin K support bone health and reduce the risk of osteoporosis.

5. Immune Function: Nutrient-dense foods provide essential vitamins and minerals that strengthen the immune system and enhance the body's ability to fight infections.

6. Brain Health: Omega-3 fatty acids from fatty fish, walnuts, and flaxseeds support brain health and cognitive function, reducing the risk of neurodegenerative diseases.

7. Digestive Health: A diet rich in fiber from nutrient-packed foods supports a healthy gut microbiome and prevents digestive issues.

8. Weight Management: Nutrient-dense foods are often lower in calories and higher in satiety-promoting nutrients, making them supportive of weight management.

Creating a Sustainable Lifestyle

1. Mindful Eating: Practice mindful eating by savoring each bite, eating slowly, and paying attention to hunger and fullness cues.

2. Culinary Exploration: Explore new recipes and cooking methods to keep meals exciting and enjoyable.

3. Social Connection: Share nutrient-packed meals and snacks with loved ones, fostering a sense of community and support.

4. Mindset Reinforcement: Continuously remind yourself of the positive impact of nutrient-packed foods on your health and well-being.

5. Celebrate Progress: Acknowledge your efforts and milestones along your journey to better health through nourishing meals and snacks.

Nutrient-packed meals and snacks are the cornerstone of a well-rounded approach to disease prevention and overall well-being. By consciously selecting foods that are rich in essential nutrients, antioxidants, and fiber, individuals can fortify their bodies against chronic diseases while enjoying enhanced energy, vitality, and vitality. Cultivating a lifestyle centered around nutrient-packed eating is a powerful investment in long-term health, providing the foundation for a fulfilling life characterized by wellness, resilience, and longevity.

•Delicious Dishes Incorporating Disease-Fighting Ingredients

The saying "you are what you eat" carries a profound truth – the foods we consume play a significant role in shaping our health and well-being. Incorporating disease-fighting ingredients into our meals is not only a proactive step toward preventing illnesses but also an opportunity to indulge in delectable flavors and textures. From vibrant vegetables and antioxidant-rich fruits to lean proteins and heart-healthy fats, the world of culinary possibilities is vast and tantalizing. In this comprehensive exploration, we dive into a variety of delicious dishes that seamlessly integrate disease-fighting ingredients, celebrating the union of health and culinary delight.

The Power of Disease-Fighting Ingredients

Disease-fighting ingredients encompass a wide array of nutrient-dense foods that are packed with vitamins, minerals, antioxidants, and phytochemicals. These components are known to have protective properties against chronic diseases, such as heart disease, diabetes, cancer, and neurodegenerative disorders. By skillfully combining these ingredients, we can create meals that not only satisfy our taste buds but also nourish our bodies from the inside out.

However, I can give you a few examples of delicious dishes that incorporate disease-fighting ingredients:

1. Rainbow Salad: Create a vibrant salad by combining a variety of colorful vegetables like spinach, bell peppers, carrots, cherry tomatoes, and purple cabbage. Top it with a dressing made from olive oil, lemon juice, and a sprinkle of turmeric for its anti-inflammatory properties.
2. Quinoa Buddha Bowl: Cook quinoa and top it with roasted sweet potatoes, steamed broccoli, sautéed kale, and avocado slices. Drizzle with a tahini dressing made from tahini, lemon juice, garlic, and a touch of maple syrup.

3. Salmon with Garlic and Ginger: Marinate salmon fillets in a mixture of minced garlic, grated ginger, soy sauce, and a dash of honey. Bake or grill until cooked through. Serve with a side of steamed vegetables for a nutritious and flavorful meal.

4. Lentil Soup: Cook lentils with onions, carrots, celery, garlic, and vegetable broth. Add turmeric, cumin, and paprika for extra flavor and anti-inflammatory benefits. Enjoy this hearty soup as a comforting and nutritious meal.

5. Berry Smoothie Bowl: Blend frozen berries, spinach, almond milk, and a scoop of protein powder for a nutrient-packed smoothie. Pour it into a bowl and top with sliced fruits, chia seeds, and granola for added texture and nutrients.

6. Chickpea Curry: Sauté onions, garlic, and ginger in a pan. Add chickpeas, diced tomatoes, and a blend of spices like turmeric, cumin, coriander, and garam masala. Simmer until the flavors meld together. Serve with brown rice or whole wheat naan bread.

7. Grilled Vegetable Skewers: Thread colorful vegetables like bell peppers, zucchini, eggplant, and cherry tomatoes onto skewers. Brush with a mixture of olive oil, lemon juice, and herbs like rosemary or thyme. Grill until tender and serve as a tasty and healthy side dish.

8. Spinach and Mushroom Stuffed Chicken Breast: Butterfly chicken breasts and stuff them with sautéed spinach, mushrooms, and garlic. Bake until the chicken is cooked through. Serve with a side of roasted vegetables for a well-rounded meal.

9. Sweet Potato and Black Bean Tacos: Roast sweet potato cubes until tender. Mash black beans with spices like cumin, chili powder, and garlic powder. Warm tortillas and spread the mashed black beans on them. Top with the roasted sweet potatoes, diced avocado, salsa, and a squeeze of lime juice for a flavorful and nutritious taco.

10. Greek Yogurt Parfait: Layer Greek yogurt with fresh berries, granola, and a drizzle of honey. Greek yogurt is rich in probiotics, which support gut health, while berries provide antioxidants and fiber. Enjoy this parfait as a healthy and satisfying breakfast or snack.

Creating a Culinary Lifestyle

Planning and Preparation:

- Meal Planning: Plan your meals ahead of time to ensure a balanced intake of disease-fighting ingredients throughout the week.
- Batch Cooking: Prepare larger quantities of ingredients like grains, proteins, and roasted vegetables to use in multiple dishes.

Seasonal Eating:

- Farmers' Market Finds: Embrace seasonal produce from local farmers' markets to enhance the flavors and nutritional content of your dishes.

Herbs and Spices:

- Flavor Boosters: Experiment with a variety of herbs and spices to add depth and complexity to your meals without relying on excessive salt or sugar.

Culinary Creativity:

- Adaptation: Modify recipes to suit your preferences while still incorporating disease-fighting ingredients.

Mindful Eating:

- Savor Every Bite: Slow down and savor the flavors, textures, and aromas of your dishes for a more satisfying eating experience.

Sharing and Enjoying:

- Social Connection: Share your disease-fighting creations with friends and family, promoting a sense of community around healthful eating.

Incorporating disease-fighting ingredients into our meals need not be a mundane task; it is an opportunity to embark on a culinary adventure that celebrates health, taste, and creativity. By embracing the vibrant world of colorful fruits, vegetables, lean proteins, and nourishing fats, we create meals that are not only delicious but also profoundly nourishing. From Mediterranean flavors to Asian inspirations, the possibilities are endless, offering a journey of culinary discovery that supports disease prevention while delighting the palate.

Chapter Ten

Case Studies: Real-Life Success Stories

•*Personal Journeys of Overcoming Illness Through Nutrition*

The transformative power of nutrition goes beyond mere sustenance; it has the potential to spark remarkable journeys of healing, recovery, and triumph over illness. Countless individuals around the world have harnessed the healing properties of food to overcome a wide range of health challenges, from chronic diseases to autoimmune disorders. These personal journeys serve as powerful testaments to the profound impact that dietary choices can have on our physical and emotional well-being. In this exploration, we delve into inspiring stories of individuals who have navigated the path of overcoming illness through the transformative force of nutrition.

Cancer Survivor's Journey: The Healing Power of Plant-Based Foods

Jennifer's journey began when she was diagnosed with breast cancer. Feeling empowered to take control of her health, she delved into extensive research on the role of nutrition in cancer prevention and treatment. Jennifer embraced a plant-based diet rich in colorful fruits, vegetables, whole grains, and legumes. These nutrient-dense foods provided her body with antioxidants, phytochemicals, and fiber that supported her immune system and aided in detoxification. Over time, Jennifer experienced increased energy levels, improved digestion, and a renewed sense of vitality. Her story underscores the potential of plant-based nutrition in supporting cancer survivors' overall well-being.

Type 2 Diabetes Reversal: Embracing Low-Glycemic Foods

John's life changed dramatically when he was diagnosed with type 2 diabetes. Frustrated by the dependence on medications, he sought an alternative approach. After consulting with a registered dietitian, he transitioned to a low-glycemic diet, focusing on whole grains, lean proteins, non-starchy vegetables, and healthy fats. By stabilizing his blood sugar levels through strategic food choices, John experienced a significant reduction in his medication dosage. His weight decreased, and he felt empowered to manage his condition naturally. John's journey illustrates how targeted dietary changes can lead to type 2 diabetes reversal and improved metabolic health.

Autoimmune Disorder Management: Harnessing Anti-Inflammatory Foods

Sarah's battle with an autoimmune disorder brought debilitating symptoms and challenges. Determined to improve her quality of life, she turned to an anti-inflammatory diet. Sarah eliminated processed foods, refined sugars, and common allergens while incorporating foods rich in omega-3 fatty acids, leafy greens, and colorful berries. The anti-inflammatory properties of these foods reduced her symptoms and provided relief from pain and inflammation. Sarah's story demonstrates the potential of nutrition in managing autoimmune disorders by modulating the body's immune response.

Heart Health Transformation: Navigating Heart Disease with a Balanced Diet

Mike's diagnosis of heart disease served as a wake-up call to prioritize his health. He embarked on a journey to reduce his risk factors through dietary changes. By reducing saturated and trans fats, Mike adopted a diet focused on lean proteins, whole grains, and heart-healthy fats. The incorporation of foods rich in soluble fiber, such as oats and legumes, helped lower his cholesterol levels. Mike's journey highlights the role of a balanced diet in supporting cardiovascular health and reducing the risk of heart-related complications.

Mental Health Recovery: The Gut-Brain Connection and Nutrient-Rich Foods

Emily's battle with anxiety and depression led her to explore the link between gut health and mental well-being. Understanding the gut-brain connection, she embraced a diet rich in prebiotics, probiotics, and nutrient-dense foods. Fermented foods, like yogurt and sauerkraut, became staples in her diet. Over time, Emily noticed improved mood, reduced anxiety, and enhanced cognitive clarity. Her story underscores the potential of nutrition in nurturing mental resilience and supporting emotional well-being.

The Impact of Support Systems and Mindset

• Community and Support: Overcoming Isolation and Navigating Dietary Changes

Tom's journey to manage his autoimmune condition was met with skepticism from his peers. However, Tom found a supportive community of individuals who shared similar health challenges. With their encouragement, he gradually adopted an anti-inflammatory diet. Connecting with others who understood his struggles provided Tom with the emotional support needed to sustain his dietary changes. His experience highlights the importance of community and shared experiences in overcoming isolation and fostering a positive mindset.

• Mindset and Resilience: Embracing Change Amidst Adversity

Sarah's battle with a chronic condition required significant lifestyle adjustments. Despite facing setbacks, she approached her dietary changes with determination and a resilient mindset. By focusing on small victories and maintaining a positive outlook, Sarah found the strength to navigate the challenges of her health journey. Her story exemplifies the transformative power of mindset in adapting to change and embracing new dietary habits.

• *Lessons Learned and Inspirational Transformations*

The power of nutrition in promoting health and well-being is a profound journey that transcends the boundaries of the plate. From preventing chronic diseases to boosting energy levels, the impact of nourishing food choices extends far beyond the immediate satisfaction of taste. Individuals around the world have harnessed the transformative potential of nutrition to achieve remarkable shifts in their physical, mental, and emotional well-being. This exploration delves into the valuable lessons learned and inspirational transformations that emerge from understanding and harnessing the power of nutrition for health.

1. The Holistic Approach to Health: Body, Mind, and Soul

The journey of harnessing the power of nutrition often reveals the interconnectedness of the body, mind, and soul. Emily's experience exemplifies this holistic perspective. Suffering from chronic fatigue and mood swings, she embarked on a journey to optimize her nutrition. As she embraced nutrient-dense foods and balanced meals, Emily noticed not only a surge in energy levels but also an improvement in her mood and mental clarity. Her story underscores that nourishing the body with the right nutrients positively impacts overall well-being, creating harmony between physical and mental health.

2. Cultivating Mindful Eating: The Art of Savoring Every Bite

The practice of mindful eating is a transformative lesson that teaches individuals to cultivate a deeper connection with their food and body. Ryan's journey illustrates this concept. Battling emotional eating and weight gain, he embarked on a path of mindfulness. By slowing down during meals, savoring each bite, and paying attention to hunger and fullness cues, Ryan developed a healthier relationship with food. His story emphasizes that mindful eating fosters a

conscious and positive connection with nutrition, promoting better digestion and overall satisfaction.

3. Healing from Within: Nutrition as a Tool for Recovery

The power of nutrition is evident in its role as a catalyst for recovery from health challenges. Laura's journey of overcoming digestive issues showcases this transformative potential. Through personalized dietary changes, Laura managed to alleviate her symptoms and regain her quality of life. The journey taught her that listening to her body's signals and making informed dietary choices played a crucial role in her healing process. Laura's story highlights the significance of using nutrition as a tool for healing and reclaiming well-being.

4. Preventing Chronic Diseases: Empowering Through Nutrient-Rich Choices

Lessons learned from personal journeys underscore that nutrition is a powerful weapon in preventing chronic diseases. Emily's story reflects this lesson. Faced with a family history of diabetes, she adopted a whole-foods, plant-based diet rich in fiber and antioxidants. As a result, Emily's blood sugar levels stabilized, and she reduced her risk of developing diabetes. Her experience illuminates that strategic dietary choices have the potential to be transformative in reducing the risk of chronic diseases.

5. Mind-Body Connection: Nutrition's Impact on Mental Health

The journey of harnessing nutrition's power extends to the realm of mental health. Daniel's experience underscores this lesson. Struggling with anxiety and low mood, he embarked on a journey to incorporate nutrient-dense foods that supported his brain health. By including omega-3 fatty acids, B vitamins, and antioxidants, Daniel noticed a significant improvement in his mood and cognitive function. His story emphasizes that nurturing the mind-body connection through nutrition can lead to remarkable transformations in mental well-being.

6. Fueling Performance and Energy: Nutrition for Active Lifestyles

The impact of nutrition is vividly demonstrated in the realm of physical performance and energy levels. Anna's journey highlights this transformational aspect. As an athlete, Anna sought to optimize her energy and endurance through nutrition. By strategically timing her meals, consuming a balanced mix of macronutrients, and staying hydrated, she experienced enhanced athletic performance and overall vitality. Anna's story emphasizes that nutrient-rich choices can serve as a source of sustainable energy and optimal physical performance.

7. Fostering Sustainable Habits: The Role of Consistency and Adaptability

Sustaining the power of nutrition for health involves adopting sustainable habits that accommodate life's dynamic nature. David's journey exemplifies this principle. Determined to lose weight and improve his well-being, he adopted a balanced eating plan that he could maintain over the long term. Rather than restrictive diets, David focused on portion control, balanced meals, and occasional indulgences. His story underscores that cultivating sustainable habits is a transformative lesson that promotes lifelong health.

8. The Joy of Culinary Exploration: Navigating Nutrient-Dense Flavors

The journey of harnessing the power of nutrition is a culinary adventure filled with diverse flavors and textures. Sarah's experience reflects this joyful exploration. Facing dietary restrictions due to health concerns, she discovered a world of nutrient-dense foods that ignited her creativity in the kitchen. By experimenting with colorful vegetables, lean proteins, and wholesome grains, Sarah found joy in crafting nourishing and delicious meals. Her story highlights that embracing nutrient-rich ingredients can lead to a culinary journey that nourishes both the body and the soul.

9. Inspiring Others Through Transformation: A Ripple Effect of Change

Inspirational transformations fueled by nutrition often have a ripple effect, inspiring others to make positive changes. Mark's journey exemplifies this transformative impact. After successfully managing his weight through dietary changes, Mark became a vocal advocate for healthy living. His story motivated friends and family to reconsider their own nutrition choices, creating a ripple effect of positive change within his community. Mark's experience underscores that individual transformations can inspire collective shifts toward healthier lifestyles.

10. Embracing Lifelong Learning: The Ever-Evolving Journey of Nutrition

The journey of harnessing nutrition's power is marked by a commitment to lifelong learning and adaptation. Julia's experience encapsulates this notion. Overcoming weight struggles, she immersed herself in nutritional education, seeking evidence-based information and experimenting with different dietary approaches. As she learned to listen to her body and adapt her choices, Julia embraced the evolving nature of her nutrition journey. Her story emphasizes that an open-minded approach to learning empowers individuals to make informed choices that support their health.

The power of nutrition in promoting health and well-being is a transformative journey rich with lessons, insights, and inspirational transformations. From holistic approaches to healing and mindful eating to preventing chronic diseases and fueling mental resilience, these journeys illustrate the potential of nutrition to positively impact every facet of life. As individuals learn to

harness the power of nutrition, they discover not only the vitality that nutrient-rich choices bring but also the profound sense of empowerment that accompanies the transformational journey toward optimal health and well-being.

Chapter Eleven

Conclusion

•*Empowering Yourself with the Knowledge of Nutritional Wellness*

In a world saturated with information about diets, superfoods, and wellness trends, understanding and harnessing the power of nutritional wellness can be both empowering and transformative. Nutritional wellness goes beyond restrictive diets and quick fixes; it's about making informed choices that nourish your body, support your well-being, and promote longevity. By equipping yourself with the knowledge of nutritional wellness, you gain the tools to navigate the complex landscape of nutrition, make sustainable dietary decisions, and cultivate a harmonious relationship with food. This exploration delves into the principles of nutritional wellness and how you can empower yourself with the knowledge to prioritize your health and thrive.

Understanding Nutritional Wellness

Nutritional wellness is a holistic approach to health that recognizes the profound impact of nutrition on the body, mind, and overall well-being. It involves making conscious choices about the foods you consume, understanding their nutritional value, and aligning your dietary habits with your health goals. Nutritional wellness is not about deprivation; it's about nourishing your body with the nutrients it needs to function optimally.

1. Educate Yourself: Building a Solid Foundation

Empowerment begins with knowledge. Educating yourself about the fundamental principles of nutrition provides a solid foundation for making informed dietary choices. Understand the essential macronutrients (carbohydrates, proteins, and fats) and micronutrients (vitamins and minerals) that your body requires for optimal functioning. Learn about the role of fiber, antioxidants, and phytochemicals in promoting health and preventing diseases.

2. Distinguish Fact from Fiction: Navigating Nutrition Myths

In the age of information, it's crucial to differentiate between evidence-based information and nutrition myths. Question sensationalized claims and fad diets, and seek information from reputable sources such as registered dietitians, medical professionals, and scientific research. Developing critical thinking skills empowers you to make choices grounded in sound nutritional science.

3. Listen to Your Body: Cultivating Intuitive Eating

Empowerment also involves tuning into your body's signals and cultivating a mindful eating practice. Intuitive eating is the practice of listening to your body's hunger and fullness cues, honoring cravings, and choosing foods that make you feel satisfied and energized. This approach fosters a healthy relationship with food and eliminates the guilt associated with eating.

4. Embrace Whole Foods: The Power of Nutrient-Rich Choices

Whole foods are the cornerstone of nutritional wellness. Incorporate a variety of colorful fruits, vegetables, whole grains, lean proteins, and healthy fats into your diet. These nutrient-dense choices provide essential vitamins, minerals, antioxidants, and fiber that support overall health and vitality.

5. Balance and Moderation: Avoiding Extremes

Nutritional wellness is about finding balance. Avoid extreme diets or restrictive approaches that can lead to nutrient deficiencies and negative relationships with food. Instead, focus on a balanced eating pattern that includes a variety of foods in moderation. Incorporate foods you enjoy while ensuring you're meeting your nutritional needs.

6. Personalization: Your Unique Nutritional Needs

Recognize that nutritional needs vary based on factors such as age, gender, activity level, and health status. Personalization is key to achieving nutritional wellness. Consult with healthcare professionals or registered dietitians to develop a dietary plan tailored to your individual needs and goals.

7. Mindful Eating: Engaging Your Senses

Mindful eating is a powerful tool in nutritional wellness. Slow down and savor each bite, engaging your senses to fully appreciate the flavors, textures, and aromas of your food. This practice enhances digestion, prevents overeating, and fosters a deeper connection with your meals.

8. Meal Planning and Preparation: Setting Yourself Up for Success

Empower yourself by planning and preparing meals ahead of time. Meal planning helps you make intentional food choices, reduces the likelihood of unhealthy impulse eating, and saves time and money. Preparing meals at home allows you to control ingredients and portion sizes.

9. Read Food Labels: Making Informed Choices

Understanding how to read food labels empowers you to make informed choices when grocery shopping. Pay attention to serving sizes, nutrient content, and ingredient lists. Aim for foods with minimal added sugars, sodium, and unhealthy fats.

10. Hydration: The Importance of Water Intake

Proper hydration is a fundamental aspect of nutritional wellness. Water supports digestion, nutrient absorption, and overall bodily functions. Carry a reusable water bottle and aim to drink water consistently throughout the day.

11. Focus on Long-Term Sustainability: Sustainable Habits

Nutritional wellness is not a short-term endeavor; it's a lifelong journey. Focus on developing sustainable habits that you can maintain over time. Avoid quick fixes or extreme diets that may yield temporary results but are difficult to maintain.

12. Seek Professional Guidance: Consulting Registered Dietitians

If you're unsure about your nutritional needs or have specific health goals, consider consulting a registered dietitian. These professionals are trained to provide evidence-based guidance tailored to your individual circumstances, ensuring that you're making choices aligned with your health objectives.

13. Celebrate Progress, Not Perfection: Positive Reinforcement

Empowerment comes from celebrating your progress rather than fixating on perfection. Recognize that nutritional wellness is about making consistent, positive choices that contribute to your overall well-being. Focus on the positive changes you're making and the impact they have on your health.

Incorporating Nutritional Wellness into Your Lifestyle

Empowering yourself with the knowledge of nutritional wellness involves integrating these principles into your daily life:

- Educate Continuously: Stay curious and committed to learning about nutrition. Read reputable books, attend workshops, and follow evidence-based resources to deepen your understanding.
- Plan and Prepare: Set aside time for meal planning, grocery shopping, and meal preparation. Having nutritious options readily available makes it easier to make healthful choices.
- Practice Mindful Eating: Engage in mindful eating practices, such as eating without distractions and paying attention to your body's hunger and fullness cues.
- Stay Hydrated: Carry a water bottle with you and aim to drink water throughout the day. Herbal teas and infused water can also contribute to hydration.
- Prioritize Whole Foods: Make whole foods the foundation of your diet. Experiment with new recipes that incorporate a variety of nutrient-rich ingredients.
- Seek Support: Surround yourself with a community that values nutritional wellness. Share your journey with friends, family, or online groups to gain support and accountability.

Empowering yourself with the knowledge of nutritional wellness is a transformative journey that places you in the driver's seat of your health. By understanding the principles of balanced nutrition, practicing mindful eating, and making informed dietary choices, you gain the tools to prioritize your well-being and cultivate a harmonious relationship with food. Through empowerment, education, and practice, you pave the way for a healthier, more vibrant, and fulfilling life.

www.ingramcontent.com/pod-product-compliance
Lightning Source LLC
Chambersburg PA
CBHW062356290526
45794CB00005B/2252